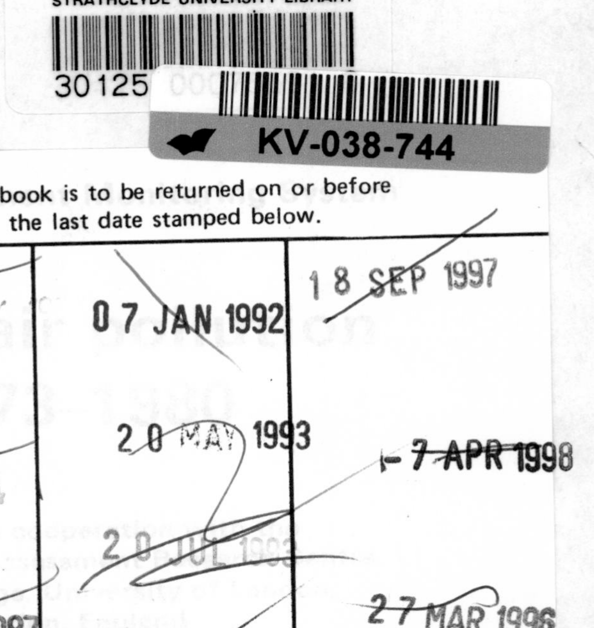


# Urban air pollution 1973–1980

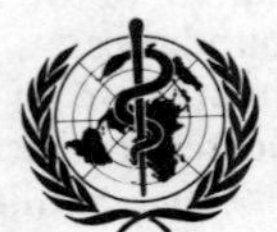

World Health Organization
Geneva
1984

ISBN 92 4 156082 7



The designations employed and the presentation of the material in this publication do not imply the expression of any opinion whatsoever on the part of the Secretariat of the World Health Organization concerning the legal status of any country, territory, city or area or of its authorities, or concerning the delimitation of its frontiers or boundaries.

The mention of specific companies or of certain manufacturers' products does not imply that they are endorsed or recommended by the World Health Organization in preference to others of a similar nature that are not mentioned. Errors and omissions excepted, the names of proprietary products are distinguished by initial capital letters.

TYPESET IN INDIA
PRINTED IN ENGLAND

83/5992—Macmillan/Spottiswoods—6000

WORLD HEALTH ORGANIZATION

# URBAN AIR POLLUTION 1973–1980

## CORRIGENDUM

Pages 69-70, Annex 3, WHO Collaborating Centres on air pollution

*Replace the list of "National Institutes and Agencies" by the following:*

Algeria – National Institute of Public Health, El Madania, Algiers
Australia – Environmental Protection Agency of Victoria, Melbourne, Victoria;
State Pollution Control Commission, Sydney, New South Wales
Belgium – Institute for Hygiene and Epidemiology, Brussels
Brazil – State Foundation for Environmental Engineering (FEEMA), Rio de Janeiro;
State Centre for Environmental and Sanitary Technology (CETESB), São Paulo
Canada – Air Pollution Control Directorate, Environment Canada, Ottawa
China – Institute of Health, Chinese Academy of Medical Sciences, Beijing
Chile – Institute for Occupational Health and Air Pollution, Santiago
Colombia – Municipal Health Department, Bogota;
Antioquia Health Service, Cali;
District Health Department, Medellín
Cuba – National Hygiene Directorate, Ministry of Public Health, Havana
Czechoslovakia – Institute of Hygiene, Prague
Denmark – National Air Pollution Laboratory, Roskilde
Egypt – Industrial Health Department, Ministry of Health, Cairo
Fiji – Ministry of Health, Suva
Finland – City Health Department, Helsinki
France – Ministry of the Environment and Quality of Life, Neuilly-sur-Seine
Germany, Federal Republic of – University Institute of Meteorology and Geophysics, Frankfurt-am-Main
Ghana – Environmental Protection Council, Accra
Greece – Environmental Pollution Control Project, Athens
Hong Kong – Air Pollution Control Unit, Department of Labour, Hong Kong
India – National Environmental Engineering Research Institute, Nagpur
Indonesia – National Institute of Health Research and Development, Ministry of Health, Jakarta
Iran (Islamic Republic of) – Environmental Health Directorate, Ministry of Health and Social Affairs, Tehran

Continued overleaf

Iraq – Ministry of Health, Baghdad
Ireland – Department of the Environment, Dublin
Israel – Division of Air Pollution and Radiation Control, Ministry of Health, Tel Aviv
Italy – Division of Air Pollution, Ministry of Health, Rome
Japan – Institute of Public Health, Tokyo
Kenya – National Public Health Laboratory, Nairobi
Kuwait – Environmental Protection Department, Al Sahab
Malaysia – Division of Environment, Ministry of Science, Technology and Environment, Kuala Lumpur
Netherlands – National Institute of Public Health, Bilthoven
New Zealand – Air Pollution Control Section, Ministry of Health, Wellington
Nigeria – Federal Ministry of Health and Social Welfare, Yaba
Pakistan – Institute of Public Health Engineering and Research, University of Engineering and Technology, Lahore
Peru – Institute for Occupational Health, Lima
Philippines – National Pollution Control Commission, Ministry of Human Settlements, Manila
Poland – Division of Sanitary Inspection, Ministry of Health and Social Welfare, Warsaw
Portugal – Laboratory for Industrial Hygiene and Air Pollution, Lisbon
Republic of Korea – Air Quality Management Bureau, Office of Environment, Seoul
Romania – Inspector General, Ministry of Health, Bucarest
Spain – Environmental Health Section, National School of Public Health, Madrid
Sri Lanka – Division of Occupational Hygiene, Labour Secretariat, Colombo
Sudan – Occupational Health Division, Ministry of Health, Khartoum
Sweden – Air Protection Laboratory, National Swedish Environment Protection Board, Nyköping
Switzerland – Health Inspector of the City of Zurich, Zurich
Thailand – Environmental Health Division, Ministry of Public Health, Bangkok
United Kingdom of Great Britain and Northern Ireland – Warren Spring Laboratory, Stevenage, Hertfordshire
United States of America – Environmental Monitoring System Laboratory, US Environmental Protection Agency, Research Triangle Park, North Carolina
Venezuela – Engineering Faculty, Central University of Venezuela, Caracas
Yugoslavia – Institute of Medical Research and Occupational Health, Zagreb

# Contents

# Preface

Following the United Nations Conference on the Human Environment, held in Stockholm in 1972, the World Health Organization established a global health-related environmental monitoring programme. This programme includes air, water, food and biological monitoring projects, all of which are also part of UNEP's Global Environment Monitoring System (GEMS).

The global air monitoring project is implemented through widespread cooperation with Member States and involves technical cooperation in air pollution measurements as well as the mutual exchange of information. The goal of the project is to monitor and understand the quality of the urban air environment and to improve the general level of public health. The air monitoring project produces biennial reports of summarized data.

The present publication, however, represents the first attempt at a complete analysis and interpretation of the urban air pollution data that have been gathered up to 1980. It aims to inform government officials and the scientific community on the concentrations of the two air pollutants most commonly associated with the combustion of fossil fuels, namely, sulfur dioxide and suspended particulate matter. The analyses have been made as comprehensive as possible in order to provide the reader with a better insight into the underlying reasons for the global phenomena observed.

The first two sections present some general information on the global air monitoring project and on the data that were available during the preparation of this publication. Following these are four sections that describe the results of the analyses. These sections include detailed statistical analyses of the complete set of data and also present in-depth analyses of some local urban situations. The comparisons with exposure limits suggested by WHO and the analysis of trends give an overview of the more common features of air pollution in many urban areas and as such attempt to present a global picture. The final part of the report contains a summary and conclusions. For details of measurement methodologies, the quality assurance procedures, and a complete data summary, the reader is referred to the annexes to this report.

# Preface

# Acknowledgements

The World Health Organization wishes to express its special thanks to Dr J. G. Kretzschmar of the Study Centre for Nuclear Energy, Mol, Belgium, who prepared the first draft; to Mr G. Akland of the Environmental Protection Agency, Research Triangle Park, NC, USA, who was involved in the compilation and analysis of the data; and to Dr B. G. Bennett of the Monitoring and Assessment Research Centre, London, England, who together with Dr H. W. de Koning, WHO, edited the final draft.

# Introduction

Air pollution in urban areas arises from a multitude of sources. The importance of a particular type of source depends to a certain extent on the location and the climate. For example, domestic heating makes a considerable contribution to air pollution in temperate regions but much less in tropical regions. On the other hand, the photochemical conversion of automobile exhaust gases into pollutants with strongly oxidizing characteristics is much more prevalent in tropical regions than in the more temperate zones. No matter where an urban area is situated, however, it will have in its atmosphere a mixture of pollutants from a variety of sources, such as heating plants (both industrial and domestic), industrial processes, waste incinerators, automobiles, and other transport vehicles. The so-called air pollution profile can vary considerably from one location to another.

The concentrations of air pollutants depend not only on the quantities that are emitted but also on the ability of the atmosphere to either absorb or disperse excess amounts. Urban areas have special characteristics in this regard. For example, they may be located in river valleys, in coastal areas, near a lake, or be surrounded by mountains. All these settings can strongly influence atmospheric dispersion characteristics and may cause distinctive pollution patterns to occur. Within cities, there are also many features that affect the concentrations of air pollutants. Examples of this are limited ventilation in the built-up or central areas of a city, and source groupings in certain areas, particularly in industrial and commercial sections, along highways, etc.

The combined effects of the source configurations and of meteorological and topographical factors are that air pollution concentrations vary over the map of an urban area. In addition, there are important temporal variations in source strengths and meteorological conditions, causing the air pollution patterns to change with different times of the day, week, or year. To measure variations in air pollution concentrations in a city, it is necessary to use a number of stations spread out over the area in question, and to make frequent or continuous measurements. To be fairly representative of the surrounding area, the air that is sampled by such stations should not be unduly affected by a nearby source. Depending on the area in which the stations are located, the sites can be classified as either industrial, commercial, or residential.

It is clear from the foregoing that as a person goes about his or her daily activities he or she will move through zones with different air pollution concentrations. The total amount of pollutants inhaled during a day constitutes the total exposure. If the exposure is high enough, it may produce either acute or immediate effects or, at lower or more persistent concentrations, chronic effects.

The exposure of urban populations in different parts of the world will vary considerably because of factors mentioned above, such as geography, climate, and type of source. Also, different life-styles and associated living conditions will contribute to widely varying human exposures to air pollution.

The WHO/UNEP air monitoring project has been designed to assess air pollution conditions on a global scale, to observe trends, and to begin to examine the relationship between pollution and human health. There are certainly problems in achieving these broad objectives. Nevertheless, it is hoped that a global view of urban air pollution can make a significant contribution towards understanding this important component of man's environment and improving the general level of public health.

# The WHO/UNEP air monitoring project

The WHO/UNEP air monitoring project was set up to assist countries in operational air pollutant monitoring, to improve the practical use of data in relation to the protection of human health, and to promote the exchange of information. The data accumulated in the network can be used to assess the air quality of urban areas throughout the world and to investigate trends in air pollution levels. This report presents an analysis of data obtained during the period 1973–1980.

## Development of the project

The air quality monitoring project was begun in 1973 by WHO. From 1973 to 1975 the project was operated on a pilot basis, during which time data reporting and handling procedures were developed and improved. The harmonization of siting, sampling, and measurement methodologies and techniques also received special attention, and a manual of selected methods of measuring air pollutants was prepared (*16*). During this first phase, 15 countries participated in the project by supplying data on sulfur dioxide ($SO_2$) and suspended particulate matter (SPM) from selected sites of their national networks. In each country, information was routinely collected from three sites of primarily industrial, commercial, and residential character, in at least one major urban area.

In 1976, the air monitoring project was expanded and included within the Global Environment Monitoring System (GEMS). Since then, financial support provided by the United Nations Environment Programme (UNEP) has been utilized to extend the network to developing countries, obtain more reliable data, and achieve an increased level of harmonization in monitoring and in data analysis and interpretation. Also in 1976, the World Meteorological Organization became a cooperating agency in the project and has since then assisted in the preparation of guidelines and in organizing workshops to train staff from developing countries (*5*). Among other international agencies participating in the project is the Commission of the European Communities (*3*), which provides the GEMS network with air monitoring data from some 40 stations operated by the member states.

The expansion of the air monitoring network took several years. Contacts were made with some 100 countries, of which 50 were visited by WHO staff or consultants to make arrangements for participation, to assist in choosing the monitoring sites, and to give practical information on the sampling and analytical techniques to be used. Sixty sets of monitoring equipment, complete with spare parts, filters, and chemicals for one year of operation, were provided and installed by experts who also trained the local staff.

After the extensive expansion and development of the network during 1976–1978, the network now changes only very slightly each year. Table 1 illustrates the growth of the network from 1973 to 1980. During this period, the number of participating countries more than doubled and the number of sites tripled. In more recent years, 25 000–30 000 daily values have been added each year to the data file for each pollutant. Not all stations report daily, since specific discontinuous sampling schemes are used at certain sites. Overall, the completeness of the data for the network as a whole has nevertheless improved with time.

Table 1. Number of countries, number of sites and number of 24-hour values in the years 1973–1980 in the WHO/UNEP air monitoring project

| Year | Number of countries | Number of sites | Number of 24-hour values[a] | |
|---|---|---|---|---|
| | | | SPM | $SO_2$ |
| 1973 | 14 | 42 | 7446 | 9936 |
| 1974 | 14 | 42 | 7263 | 8833 |
| 1975 | 15 | 44 | 10839 | 13831 |
| 1976 | 23 | 97 | 20773 | 24874 |
| 1977 | 27 | 101 | 27525 | 31448 |
| 1978 | 30 | 106 | 25651 | 27760 |
| 1979 | 34 | 146 | 29986 | 33770 |
| 1980 | 33 | 136 | 25408 | 29135 |

[a] Hourly values were aggregated to form 24-hour averages where appropriate.

The geographical coverage of the network at the end of 1980 is illustrated by the map in Fig. 1. It may be noted that the coverage is better in the northern hemisphere where a number of industrialized countries supply an important number of data from their national, regional, and local networks. Since most of the sites in the developing countries became operational after 1976, fewer data are available from these locations.

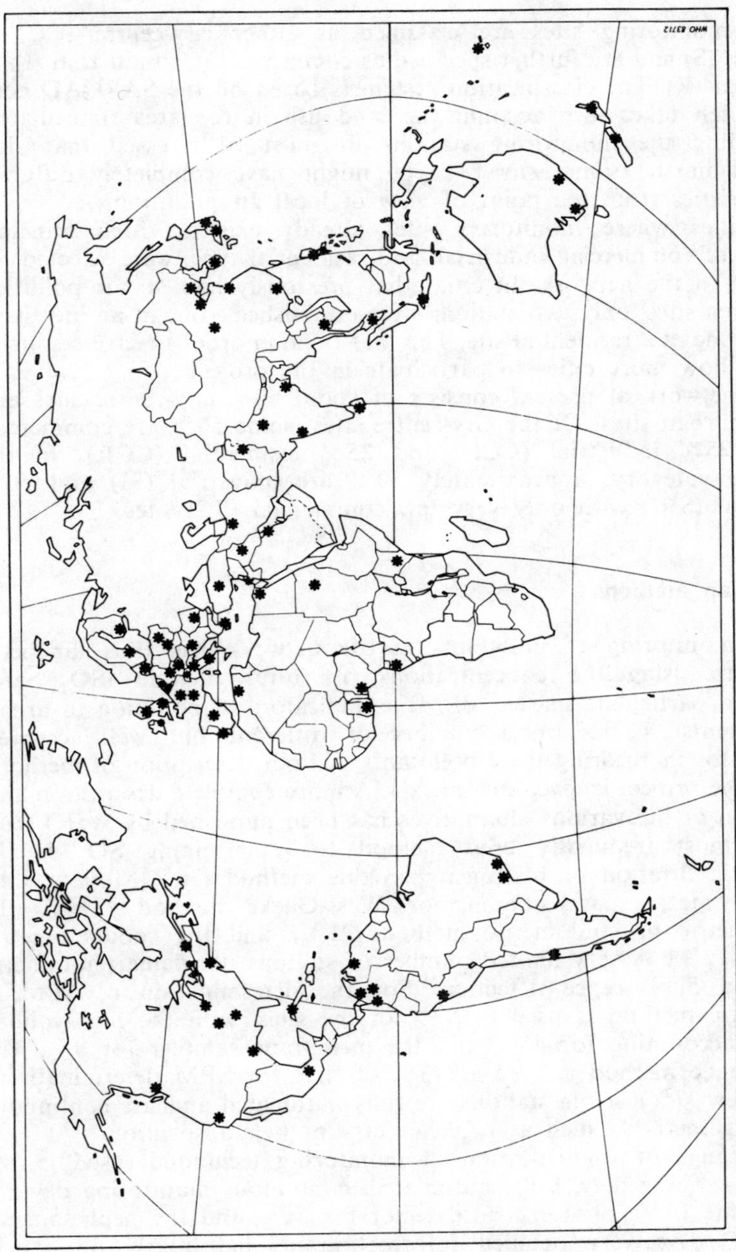


Fig. 1. Monitoring locations of the WHO/UNEP air monitoring project at the end of 1980

## Monitoring sites

The monitoring sites are classified as either city-centre (CC) or suburban (S) and are further specified as commercial (C), industrial (I), or residential (R). The classification system is based on the SAROAD code (*23*), which takes into account the land use in the area immediately surrounding the monitoring stations. It must be stressed that sites classified in the same way by type might have completely different characteristics from the point of view of local air pollution.

In cities where monitoring sites already existed, three principal stations, of commercial, industrial, and residential type, were selected for inclusion in the network. In cities that previously had no air pollution monitoring sites, only two stations were established—one at an industrial site and one at a residential site. This was done in order to save resources and to allow more cities to participate in the project.

The network at present consists of about 60% city-centre sites and 40% suburban sites. Of the city-centre sites, some 50% are commercial (CCC), 25% industrial (CCI), and 25% residential (CCR). In the suburban category, approximately 50% are industrial (SI) and 50% residential (SR), with only very few commercial (SC) sites.

## Monitoring methods

The monitoring of pollutants in the network has thus far been limited to using the concentrations of sulfur dioxide ($SO_2$) and suspended particulate matter (SPM) as indicators of pollution in urban environments. There are a number of different but well accepted methods for monitoring these pollutants. A brief description of methods used in the project is given in Annex 1. A more complete description and discussion of the various alternatives has been published by WHO (*16*).

The most frequently used method for determining $SO_2$ is the acidimetric titration or hydrogen peroxide method (36%), followed by the colorimetric pararosaniline or West-Gaeke method (27%), the amperometric or coulometric method (21%), and the conductometric method (12%). A very limited number of stations use flame photometry or pulsed fluorescence detection. For the determination of SPM, a gravimetric method is used at 50% of the sites, with the high-volume sampler accounting for 46% and the membrane sampler for 4%. The smoke-shade method is used at 43% of sites for SPM determinations. Only a few (7%) of the stations are fully automated and use continuous measuring methods such as nephelometry or beta-absorption.

The range of sophistication of monitoring techniques used in the network varies widely. Fully automated, continuous monitoring devices, such as the flame photometric detector for $SO_2$, and the nephelometer for SPM, give very detailed information, as half-hourly or hourly outputs, on the temporal variation in the measured levels. Commonly used manual techniques, such as the hydrogen peroxide method for $SO_2$ and the smoke measurement technique for SPM, do not provide this temporal resolution, since they integrate sampling over 24 hours. This information is adequate for the network, however, and is very useful in studying weekly cycles, seasonal influences and trends, and for making comparisons with air quality criteria or standards.

To overcome difficulties with the interpretation of data produced by different measuring techniques, comparison stations have been set up at various sites in the network. Different equipment is operated in parallel for limited periods. In addition to these field experiments, some inter-laboratory comparison studies for $SO_2$ have also been undertaken. Quality assurance is an important part of any monitoring network. Additional details of the quality assurance for the GEMS air monitoring project are given in Annex 2.

## Project implementation

The air monitoring project is implemented through the WHO Regional Offices, where operational contacts with the national agencies and institutes participating in the project are established and maintained. In each of the participating countries, a government agency or institution (national centre) is identified as the focal point for carrying out the project in that country. In addition, a number of WHO Collaborating Centres assist in project implementation by providing consultants, conducting quality assurance exercises, operating the data bank, and preparing data reports. Extensive support is provided by the Environmental Monitoring and Systems Laboratory of the Environmental Protection Agency, Research Triangle Park, USA, which operates the data bank and assists in the production of data reports for the project. A complete list of the WHO Collaborating Centres and the national agencies and institutes is given in Annex 3.

# Data presentation

## Statistical summaries

Daily $SO_2$ and SPM concentration measurements produce large amounts of data which are best managed and reported after statistical analysis. It is most convenient to summarize annual sets of daily measurements for each site in a cumulative frequency table and in corresponding cumulative frequency plots.

The annual statistics for each pollutant at each site in the air monitoring network have been published in biennial reports (*17*, *18*, *20*, *22*). An illustration of the format in which the data are presented is given in Table 2. This table shows the summary of $SO_2$ concentrations at the city-centre commercial site in Tokyo and gives the number of valid measurements made during the year. In this example, the records are fairly complete, with no more than 11 days missing in any one year. The minimum and maximum recorded daily averages and the percentiles of the cumulative frequency distribution are also given. Finally, the arithmetic and geometric means, and standard deviations are listed.

## Data completeness and representativeness

Not all stations have reported data with sufficient completeness to allow representative annual variables (means, percentiles etc.) to be determined. A distinction must be made between data sets that are incomplete because a discontinuous sampling scheme was intentionally selected, e.g., one measurement every five days, and data sets that are incomplete despite all efforts and precautions. The former, if properly planned, provide representative annual values. The latter require individual evaluation to judge the representativeness of each set.

Loss of data may be due to malfunctioning or breakdown of sampling or measuring devices, to elimination of questionable data before recording, or to errors during transfer or processing of data. Representativeness of the available data set depends on the nature of the problem and on the distribution of valid data. If, for instance, some 15%

Table 2. Daily averages of sulfur dioxide concentrations ($\mu g/m^3$) recorded at the city-centre commercial site, Tokyo, 1973–1980[a]

| Year | Number of values (n) | Minimum value | Percentile | | | | | | | | | Maximum value | Arith-metic mean | SD | Geo-metric mean | SD |
|---|---|---|---|---|---|---|---|---|---|---|---|---|---|---|---|---|
| | | | 10 | 30 | 50 | 60 | 70 | 80 | 90 | 95 | 98 | | | | | |
| 1973 | 363 | LD[b] | 38 | 55 | 70 | 75 | 83 | 94 | 108 | 122 | 140 | 149 | 71 | 28 | 65 | 1.6 |
| 1974 | 363 | LD | 44 | 57 | 68 | 72 | 78 | 85 | 93 | 106 | 118 | 152 | 68 | 21 | 65 | 1.4 |
| 1975 | 363 | LD | 38 | 53 | 64 | 68 | 75 | 80 | 91 | 104 | 124 | 186 | 65 | 23 | 60 | 1.5 |
| 1976 | 366 | LD | 42 | 52 | 63 | 68 | 73 | 81 | 92 | 107 | 118 | 210 | 66 | 23 | 62 | 1.4 |
| 1977 | 358 | LD | 45 | 58 | 68 | 76 | 79 | 84 | 92 | 97 | 110 | 144 | 68 | 20 | 64 | 1.5 |
| 1978 | 364 | LD | 34 | 47 | 52 | 58 | 60 | 65 | 76 | 84 | 100 | 123 | 54 | 18 | 51 | 1.5 |
| 1979 | 363 | LD | 37 | 52 | 55 | 58 | 60 | 65 | 73 | 81 | 102 | 183 | 56 | 18 | 53 | 1.4 |
| 1980 | 355 | LD | 37 | 50 | 55 | 58 | 60 | 63 | 71 | 79 | 97 | 126 | 55 | 17 | 51 | 1.5 |

[a] The conductometric method is used at this site.
[b] LD = lower than detection limit (here 26 $\mu g\ SO_2/m^3$).

of the data is missing, and the missing data are distributed evenly and somewhat randomly over the year, the data set can be accepted as being representative for the entire year. There remains the possibility, however, that the extreme values (maximum or minimum) have not been recorded. If, on the other hand, the missing 15% of the data is grouped, e.g., almost two consecutive months without reported values, the representativeness of the data set for the year is doubtful, especially when important seasonal changes have been noted for the site. If the temporal variability of the daily levels is small, the consequences of a prolonged loss of data could be minimal.

## Data set for the network

A summary of the yearly statistics for each pollutant at each site is given in Annex 4. The table which constitutes Annex 4 lists the number of measurements recorded in the year, the mean, maximum, and 98th percentile value, by country and city. Whenever a data set is judged as not being representative of the entire year, it is marked with an asterisk. These data must be disregarded or used with great care in subsequent analyses.

There are 1451 data sets entered in Annex 4, each set consisting of $SO_2$ or SPM concentration values at a specific site for a specific year. The data cover the period 1973–1980. There are 736 $SO_2$ and 715 SPM listings (368 high-volume sampler, 299 smoke determination, 40 membrane gravimetric sampler, and 8 beta-attenuation method). Of these, 74% of the $SO_2$ sets and 79% of the SPM sets are judged to be representative. The range of values, means, various comparisons, and interpretation of the data set are presented in subsequent chapters.

## Graphical representations

Although the tabular presentation of data, as in Table 2 and Annex 4, is very convenient for summarizing and transmitting information, more insight into the data can be gained by graphical illustrations. It is generally recognized that the yearly sets of daily measurements are best represented by log-normal distributions (*21*). Within acceptable limits, the data form straight line plots on log-normal graph paper.

Although not ideal, this approach is certainly the most pragmatic one, especially when based on the values in the range from the median to the 98th percentile, this being the most interesting range from the perspective of health-related air monitoring. In the majority of the data sets, the lowest values are close to or even below the detection limit so that their accuracy is questionable and their real value quite often unknown. At the other end of the distribution, the representativeness and accuracy of the highest concentrations of the pollutant are quite often hard to evaluate.

Errors due to sampling, faulty instruments or erroneous reporting or analysis are frequent. Furthermore, local and exceptional phenomena may also explain certain extreme values.

## Examples of log-normal presentations

Examples of the log-normal cumulative frequency distribution plots are illustrated in Fig. 2. These show $SO_2$ concentrations at the three sites in Tokyo and Zagreb in 1973 and in 1980. The data points are indicated at regular, usually ten percentile, intervals. The straight lines have been drawn through the 50th and 95th percentile points. The slopes of the lines indicate the temporal variability. High variability is generally due to pronounced seasonal changes in the concentrations of the pollutants.

In the example of Tokyo in Fig. 2, the small slopes of the cumulative frequency distribution curves illustrate the low variability in the measured daily $SO_2$ concentrations. Both variability and absolute concentrations decreased from 1973 to 1980 in approximately the same way for all three sites. The city-centre industrial (CCI) site showed the highest $SO_2$ pollution level, while the suburban residential (SR) site had the lowest level.

In the example of Zagreb, the straight lines fit the data adequately, especially in the 50th–98th percentile range. The steep slopes indicate greater variability due to important seasonal influences.

Plots of the monthly average $SO_2$ values given in Fig. 3 illustrate the seasonal variability. A comparison of the 1980 data for the city-centre commercial site in Tokyo with the 1973 data shows that some higher concentrations have been reduced, but there is little apparent variation during different seasons. The longer-term monthly averages show higher $SO_2$ concentrations in the winter months at the industrial site and more recognizable seasonal variations at the residential site.

The monthly $SO_2$ data from Zagreb show a much more pronounced seasonal variation, which has been somewhat reduced from 1973 to 1980 at the city-centre commercial site. The plots of longer-term averages in Fig. 3 show evident seasonal variations at all of the Zagreb sites. It is interesting to note that, in 1973, unusually marked changes in ambient $SO_2$ concentrations occurred during the months between January and April and September and December. This explains the bimodal distribution seen for that year for the data from the city-centre commercial site at Zagreb (see Fig. 2). In 1980, however, owing to local emission abatement, the extreme values were much reduced and there was much less seasonal variation (Fig. 3).

Another example of the way in which unusual source emissions and meteorological conditions can affect the cumulative frequency distribution is the data set from the city-centre commercial site in London. Most of the daily $SO_2$ and smoke concentrations are very well approximated by the straight line log-normal plots, illustrated in Fig. 4.

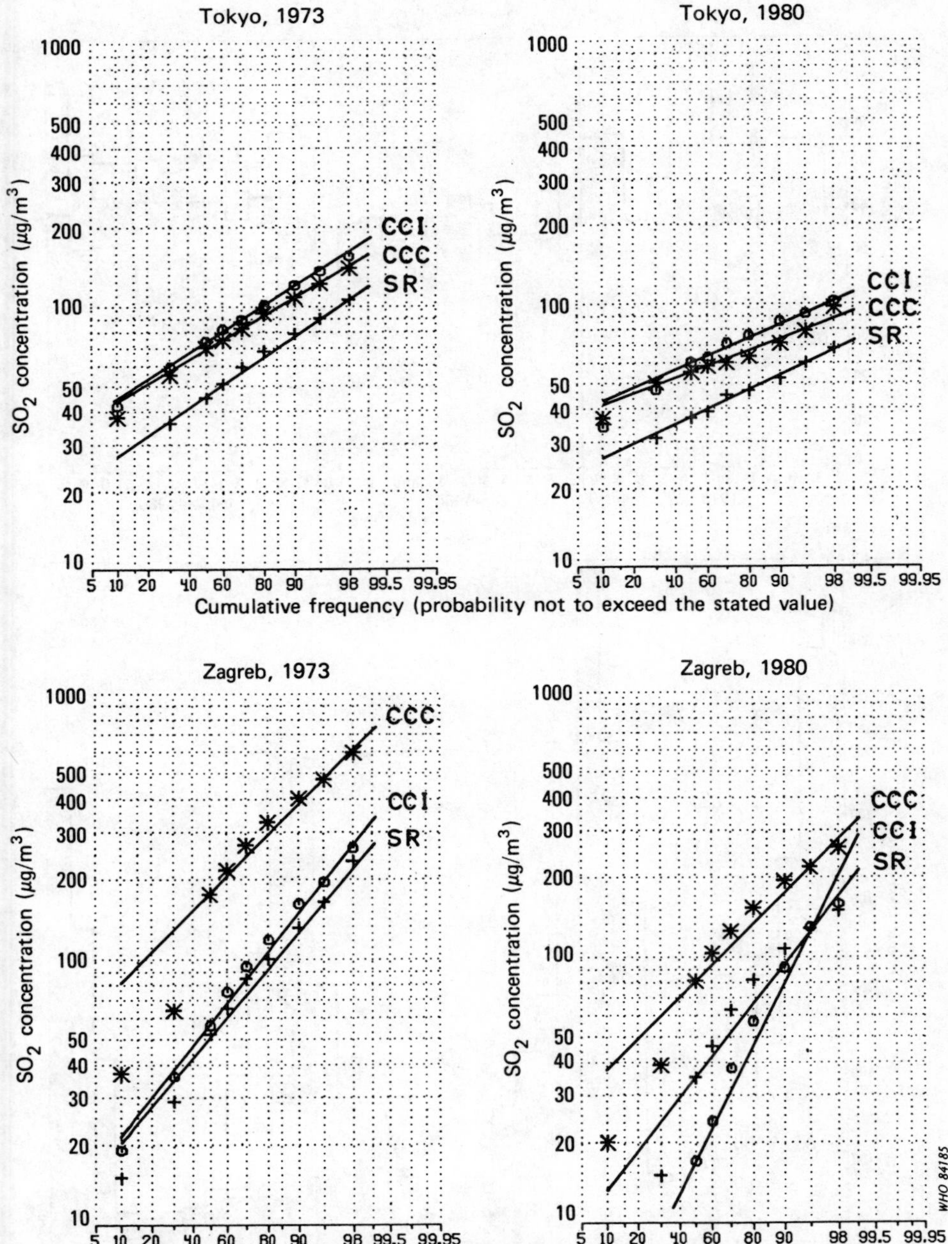


Fig. 2. Cumulative frequency distributions of daily $SO_2$ concentrations in Tokyo and Zagreb at city-centre commercial (CCC), city-centre industrial (CCI), and suburban residential (SR) sites

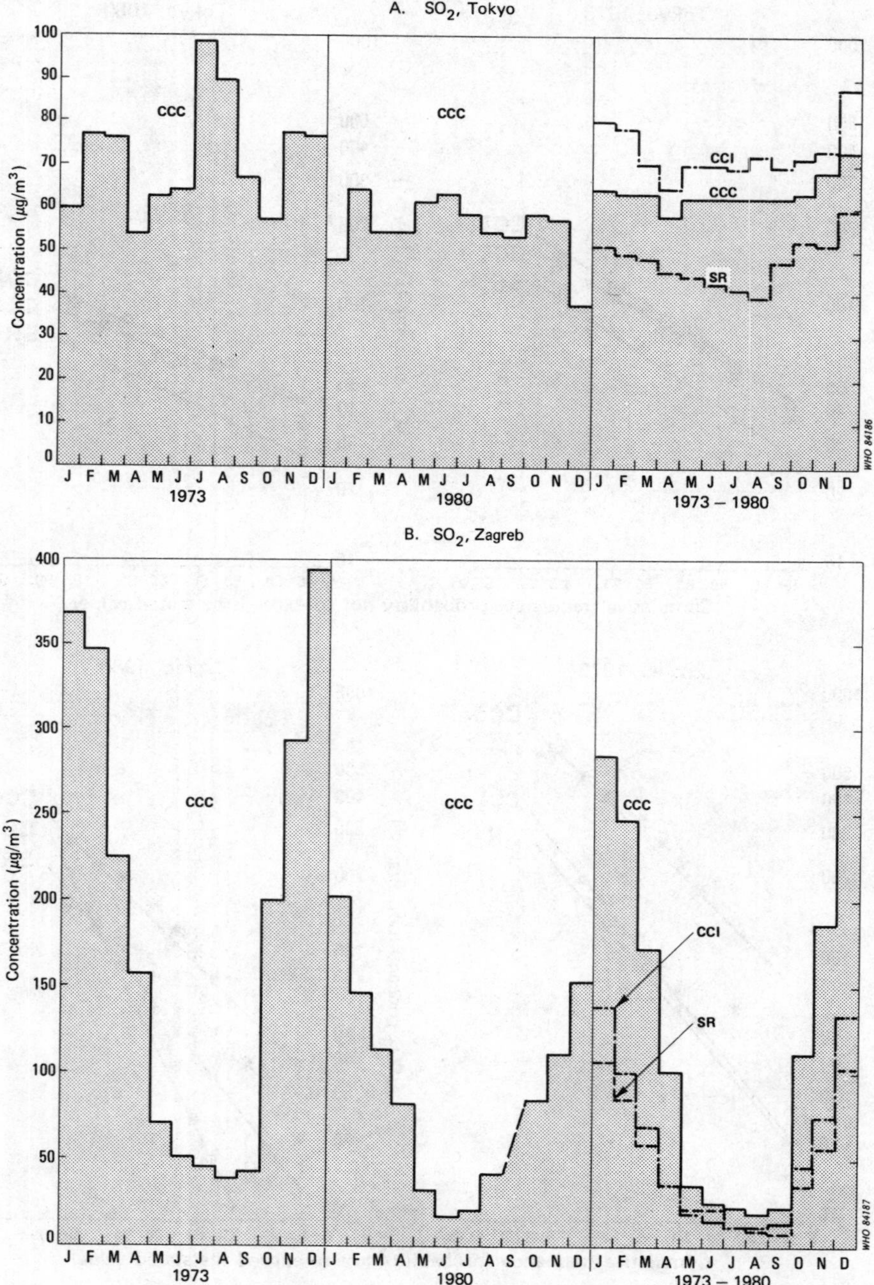


Fig. 3. Monthly variations of $SO_2$ concentrations in Tokyo (A) and Zagreb (B) at city-centre commercial (CCC), city-centre industrial (CCI) and suburban residential (SR) sites

Even the observed maxima are generally almost correctly indicated by the log-normal plot, e.g., smoke in 1974 and 1979, and $SO_2$ in 1974. The observed maximum daily average $SO_2$ concentration in 1979 is somewhat above the line, probably due to the abnormally high $SO_2$ concentrations in January and February 1979—two of the coldest months of the past 20 years—with correspondingly high energy consumption for heating during that period.

In Fig. 4, the maxima for $SO_2$ and smoke in 1975 at this London site lie above the line drawn through the 50th and 95th percentile points. The observed maximum for $SO_2$ was 840 $\mu g/m^3$ against 670 $\mu g/m^3$ approximated from the line, and for smoke 430 $\mu g/m^3$ against an estimated value of 200 $\mu g/m^3$. An explanation for these abnormally high values is that in December 1975, there was a period of adverse meteorological conditions (persistent, low, stable temperatures and low winds) during which there was poor dispersion of pollutants (*1*). And since the temperatures were unusually low, more heating was used during that period, causing the worst pollution conditions since 1962. The daily records for $SO_2$ and smoke for 1975 (Fig. 5) highlight the exceptional character of the observed concentrations during that period.

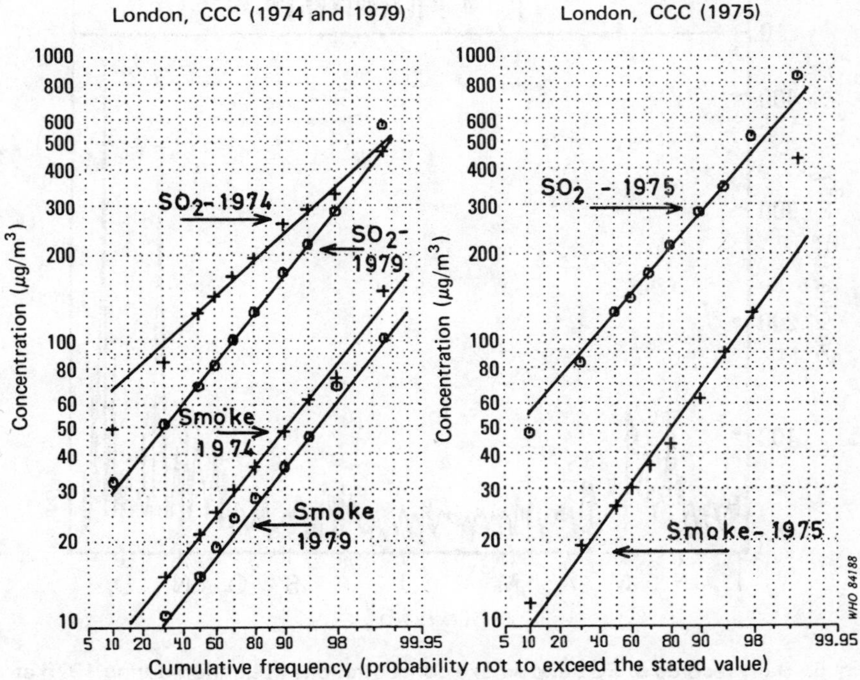


Fig. 4. Cumulative frequency distributions of daily $SO_2$ concentrations in London at the city-centre commercial (CCC) site

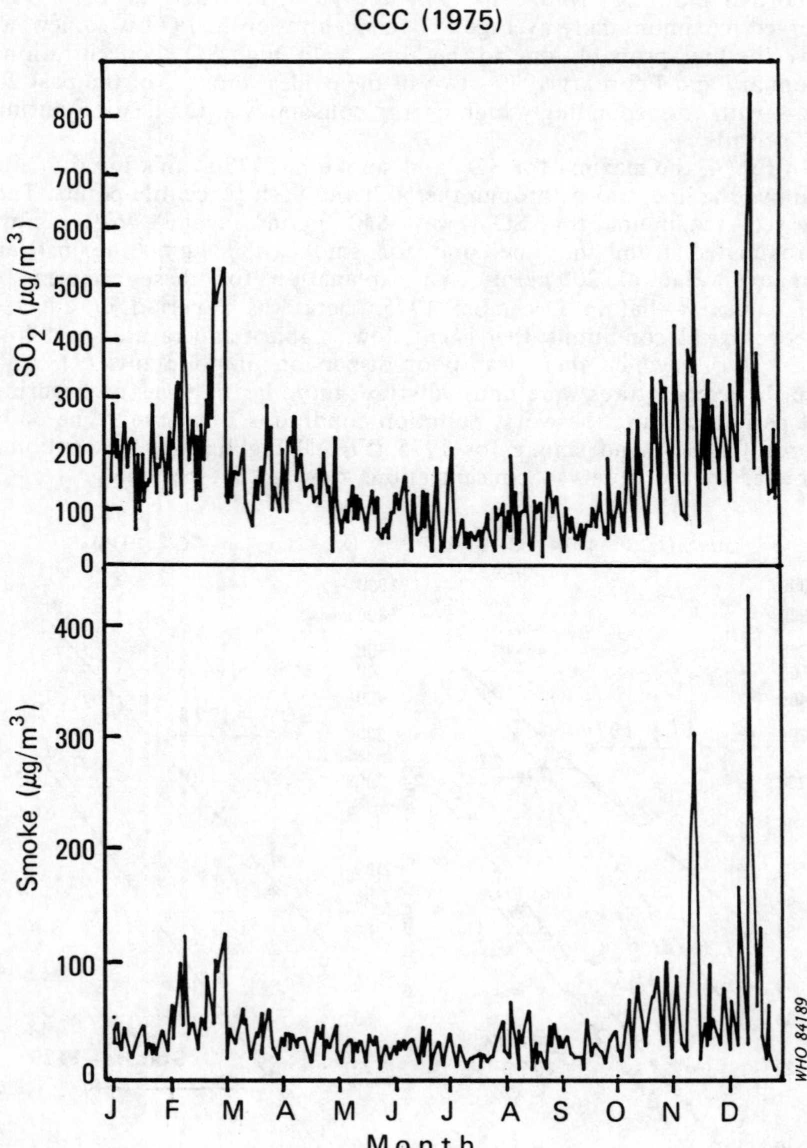


Fig. 5. Daily records of $SO_2$ and smoke concentrations in London during 1975 at the city-centre commercial (CCC) site

The above examples illustrate some of the difficulties that may be encountered in fitting straight lines to the cumulative frequency distribution. Generally, further local information concerning, for example, seasonal variations in emission patterns and pollution episodes, may help in interpreting the significance of the points deviating from the fitted lines.

# Analysis of basic variables

The operation of the GEMS air monitoring network has resulted in the acquisition of a substantial amount of data on the air quality of urban areas. There are many ways of analysing these data. The basic approach is to look at each pollutant at each site in each year. But more encompassing views can also be taken, for example, by examining values for particular variables for a pollutant from all sites, or from specific types of site. Analyses can also be made for annual mean values and extreme values (usually the 98th percentiles or the maxima).

## Global variations

It may be useful first to take a more pictorial view of the data. The longer-term mean values of pollutant concentrations in urban areas of the GEMS air monitoring project are shown in Fig. 6, 7, and 8. To minimize the year to year variations, the period 1975–1980 has been taken for illustration. Results are given for two sites in each city. Where more than two sites were operational, the lowest and highest reported values are shown, giving an indication of the spatial variability of the pollutant concentrations within the city.

It may be seen from Fig. 6 that $SO_2$ concentrations tend to be low to intermediate in Australia, Canada, New Zealand, and the USA. Higher values are reported at some sites in Europe, South America, and Asia. Fig. 7 and 8 show the different preferences for methods to determine suspended particulate matter (SPM). The high-volume, gravimetric method is used in North America, Europe, Asia, and Australia. Smoke concentrations are measured in Europe, South America and New Zealand. The higher SPM concentrations at sites in south-west Asia and India may be due to dust in the air, not necessarily of anthropogenic origin or of respirable size. A more specific interpretation would require additional information on the local emission sources and environmental conditions.

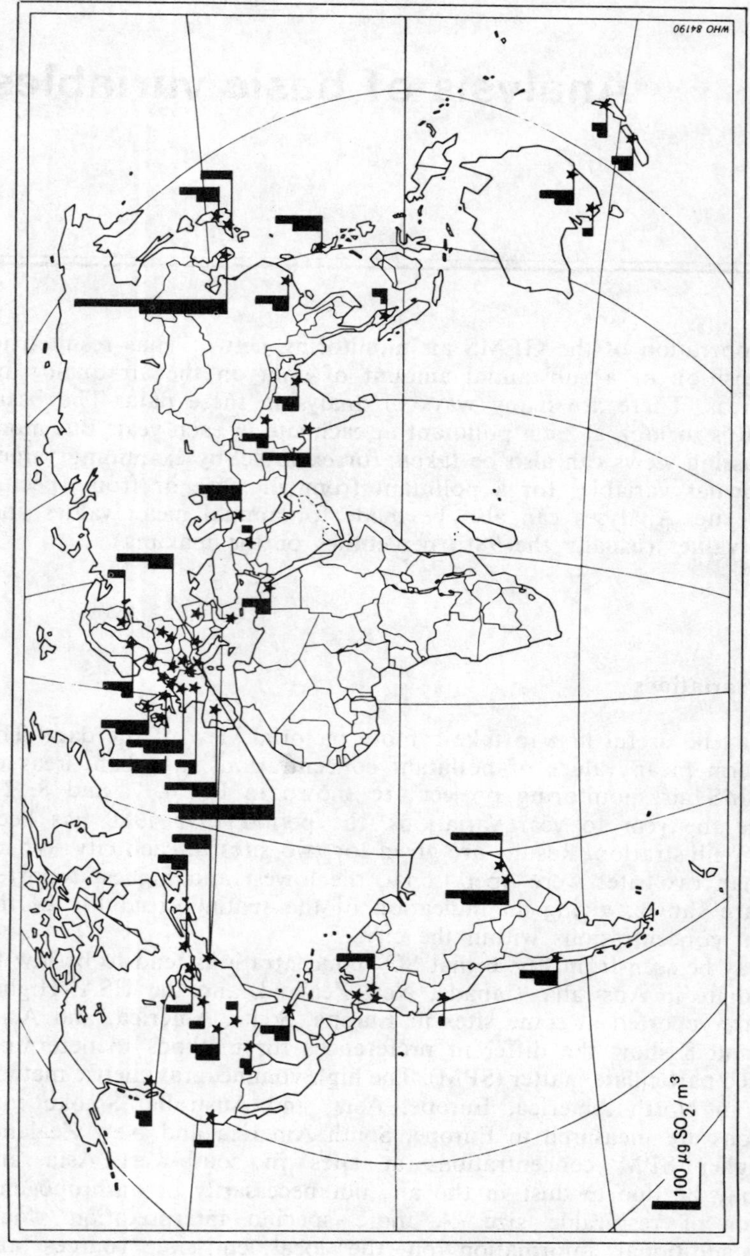


Fig. 6. Average $SO_2$ concentrations for 1975–1980 in cities of the GEMS project (the highest and lowest averages are indicated for cities with more than two sites; otherwise, results are given for the existing sites)

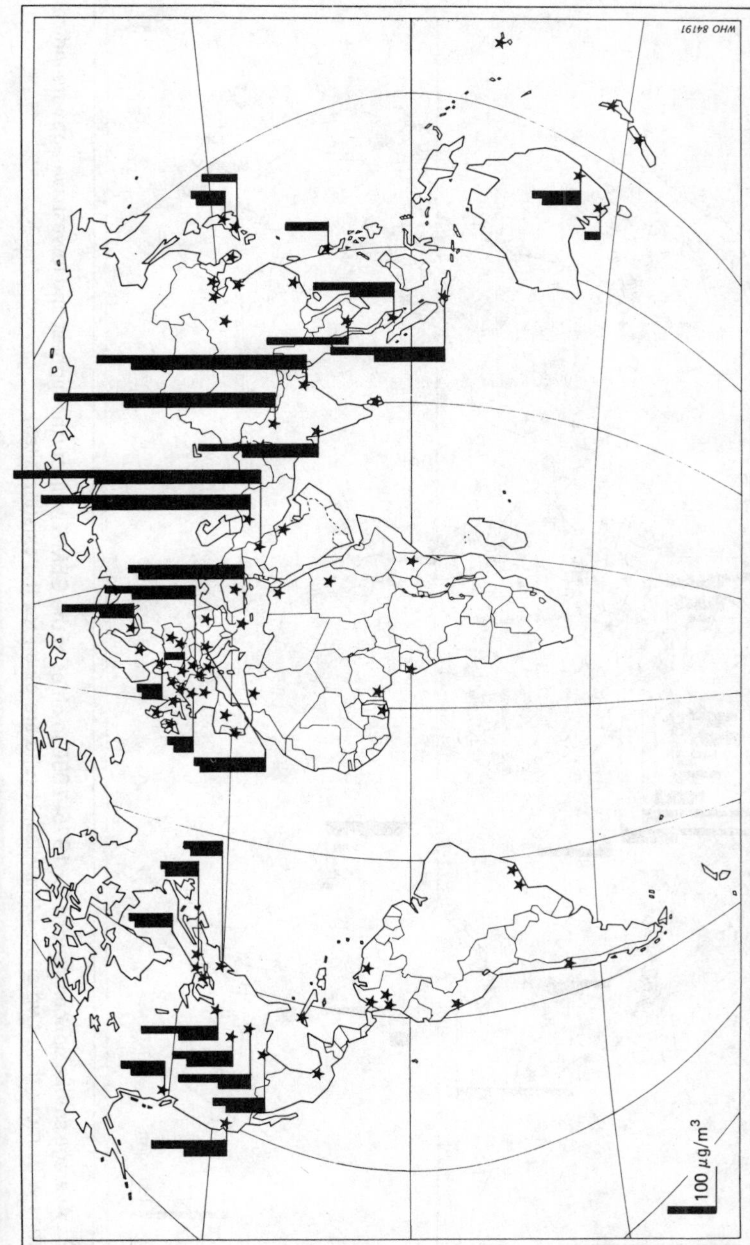


Fig. 7. Average SPM (gravimetric method) concentrations for 1975–1980 in cities of the GEMS project (the highest and lowest averages are indicated for cities with more than two sites; otherwise, results are given for the existing sites)

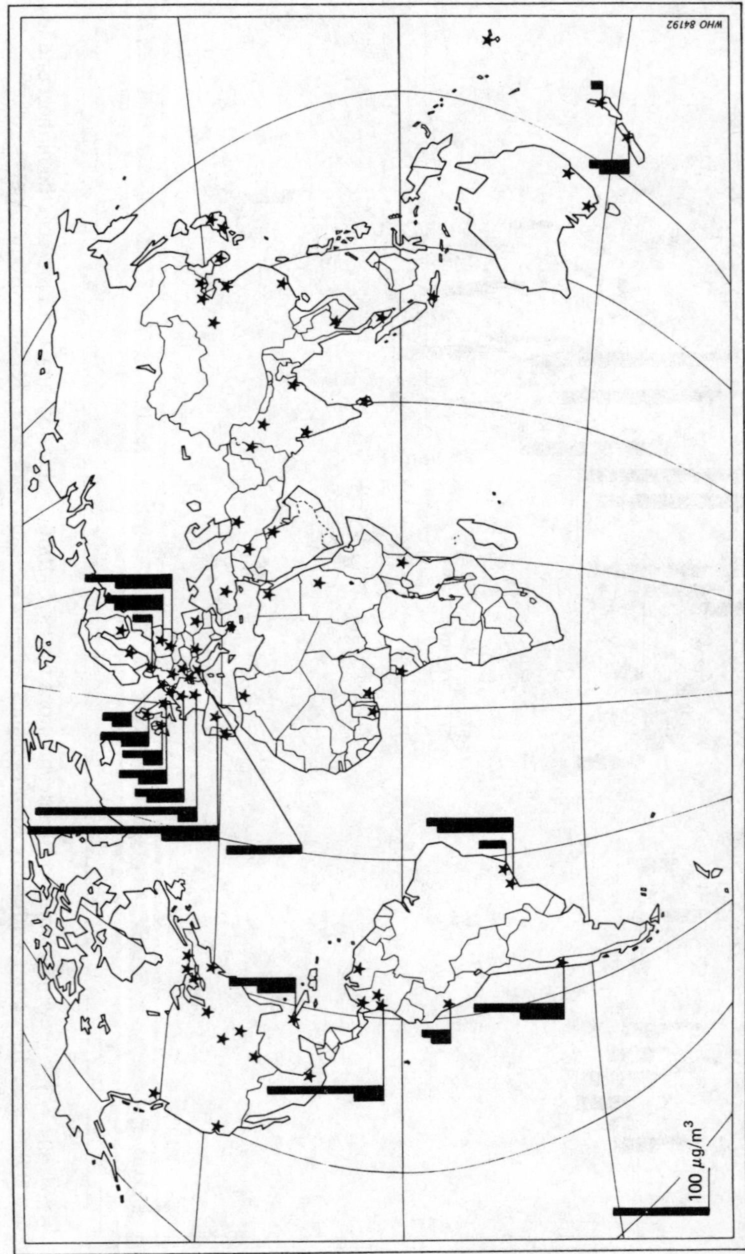


Fig. 8. Average smoke concentrations for 1975–1980 in cities of the GEMS project (the highest and lowest averages are indicated for cities with more than two sites; otherwise, results are given for the existing sites)

## Distribution of annual mean values

Comprehensive analyses of the GEMS data reported in Annex 4 are given below. Continuing with overall views of the data, Fig. 9, 10, and 11 show the annual mean values obtained by various measurement methods for $SO_2$ and SPM (high-volume and smoke determinations) acquired from all sites over the entire period of the project (1973–1980). For each pollutant, the distribution of values peaks in the lower range with long tailing out to the upper range. The distribution of annual average concentrations at all sites appears approximately log-normal, in a similar way to the distributions of daily average values at individual sites.

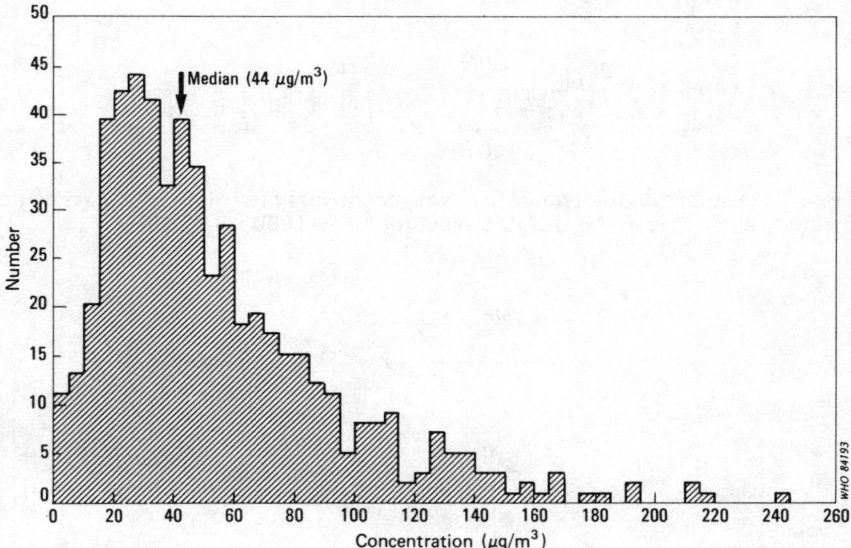


Fig. 9. Distribution of annual average concentrations of $SO_2$ at all sites of the GEMS project for 1973–1980

For $SO_2$ (Fig. 9), the range of representative annual mean concentrations is from 3 $\mu g/m^3$ to 242 $\mu g/m^3$. There are 4 values from two city-centre sites in Milan which are greater than 200 $\mu g/m^3$. At the other extreme, with annual means $\leqslant 5$ $\mu g/m^3$, though with some incompleteness in reported data, are sites in Hong Kong, Houston and Harris (Texas), Kuala Lumpur, Lima, Melbourne, and Toulouse. Most of the sites (90%) are within the range 11–135 $\mu g/m^3$. The central range for 50% of the values is 27–72 $\mu g/m^3$. The median for all $SO_2$ data is 44 $\mu g/m^3$.

For suspended particulate matter determined by the high-volume

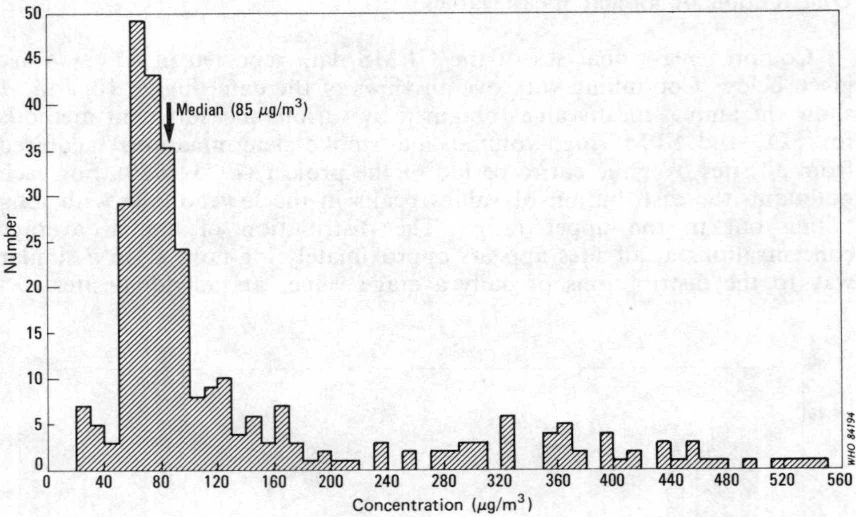


Fig. 10. Distribution of annual average concentrations of SPM (gravimetric method) at all sites of the GEMS project for 1973–1980

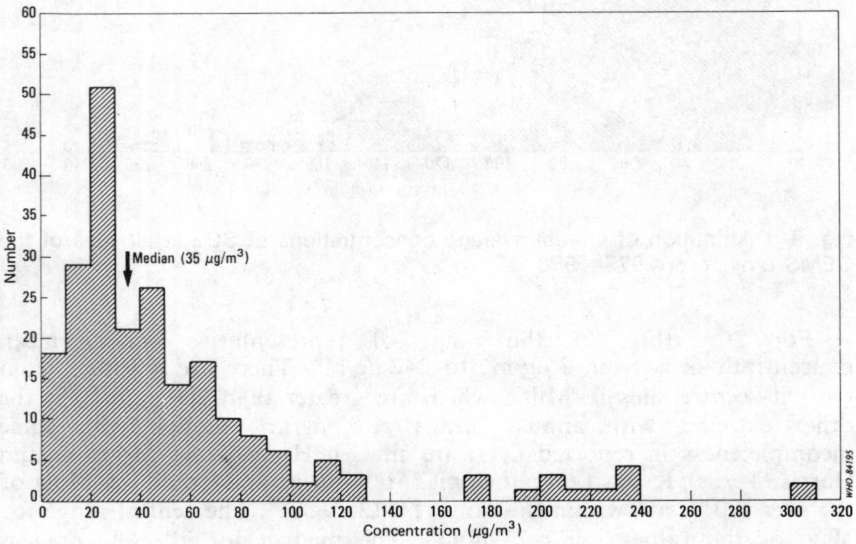


Fig. 11. Distribution of annual average concentrations of smoke at all sites of the GEMS project for 1973–1980

sampling method (Fig. 10), the range is 24–547 $\mu g/m^3$. There is a long tail of measurements above 200 $\mu g/m^3$, amounting to 55 of the 303 data points. Three cities, Calcutta, Delhi, and Tehran, account for the 40 points above 300 $\mu g/m^3$. At the low end of the range are 12 annual means less than 40 $\mu g/m^3$, at Copenhagen and Melbourne. The range for 90% of all values is 49–413 $\mu g/m^3$, and for the central 50% of the data, 67–142 $\mu g/m^3$. The median SPM (high-volume) value is 85 $\mu g/m^3$.

The range of the 225 values for SPM determined as smoke (Fig. 11) is 4–307 $\mu g/m^3$. Only two cities, Madrid and Tehran, reported annual averages greater than 200 $\mu g/m^3$. Most smoke values are tightly bunched in the lower range ($< 130\ \mu g/m^3$). The range for 90% of the values is 6–196 $\mu g/m^3$, and for the central 50% of the data, 22–66 $\mu g/m^3$. The median value for smoke is 35 $\mu g/m^3$.

The log-normal plots of the cumulative frequency distributions of the annual average concentration values of the 1973–1980 data sets are illustrated in Fig. 12. The figure shows the plots for each pollutant at all sites, for city-centre and suburban sites, and for industrial, commercial, and residential sites. There is not a great deal of difference in these separate designations. In general, the suburban and residential sites report lower pollution levels than the commercial, industrial, and city-centre sites.

## Distribution of maximum values

The 98th percentile ($P_{98}$) values presented in Annex 4 are representative of the maximum daily concentrations. In particular, the $P_{98}$ value corresponds to the concentration that is not exceeded for more than 7 days during the year. The distributions of these values are shown in Fig. 13. There are similarities between types of site as compared with the annual means. The central values for all sites (50th percentile point in the $P_{98}$ plots) are approximately 140 $\mu g/m^3$ for $SO_2$, 190$\mu g/m^3$ for SPM (high-volume) and 130 $\mu g/m^3$ for smoke.

## Distribution of geometric standard deviation

An additional parameter which can be examined in the entire data set is the geometric standard deviation ($\sigma_g$). This is the slope of the log-normal plot and is an indication of the variability of pollutant concentrations at the various sites. Variability is usually most strongly influenced by seasonal variations in source emissions and meteorological conditions.

The distributions of $\sigma_g$ values are shown in Fig. 14, combining the information from all of the sites. The shapes of the distributions are nearly identical for each pollutant at the various sites: city-centre, suburban, commercial, industrial, residential. The distributions for $SO_2$ and smoke are strikingly similar and are quite different from that for

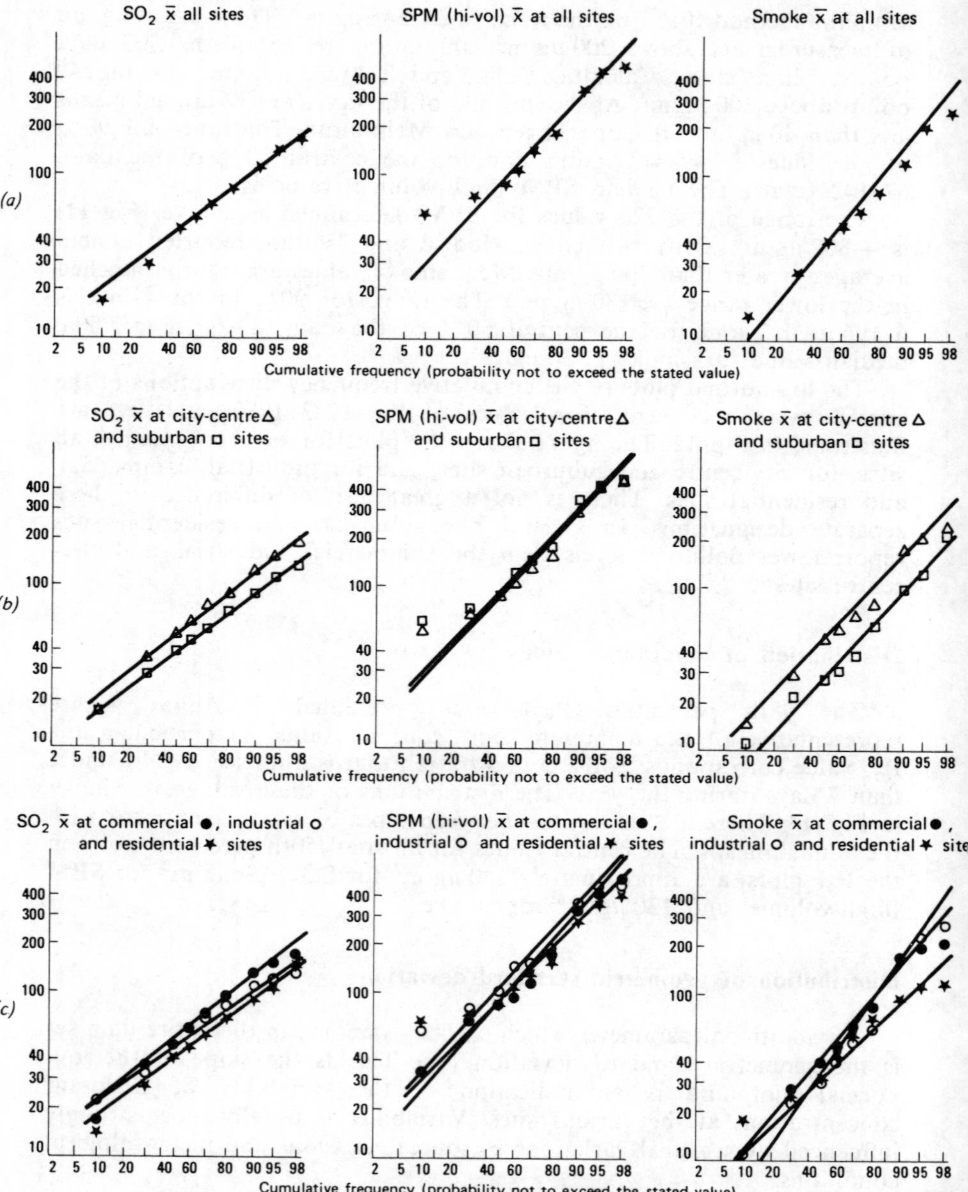


Fig. 12. Cumulative frequency distributions of annual average concentrations ($\bar{x}$) of $SO_2$, SPM (gravimetric method), and smoke for 1973–1980, (*a*) at all sites, (*b*) at city-centre (CC), and suburban (S) sites, and (*c*) at commercial (C), industrial (I), and residential (R) sites

the SPM (high-volume) measurements. The average value of $\sigma_g$ for $SO_2$ and smoke measurements is between 2.0 and 2.2, while the variability for high-volume measurements is on average much less, with the average $\sigma_g$ being around 1.6. The range of $\sigma_g$ is also significantly larger for $SO_2$ and smoke than it is for the high-volume SPM measurements. There are a limited number of high $\sigma_g$ values which occur at certain sites, especially for smoke.

The unusually high variation in the concentrations of smoke at Christchurch, New Zealand, is shown in Fig. 15. Variability at residential, commercial, and industrial sites is similar, but smoke is much more variable than $SO_2$. It can be shown in further analyses that smoke concentrations significantly increase as soon as the outside temperature drops below 10°C. During the coldest months, monthly average smoke concentrations are approximately three times the annual average. The maximum daily concentrations reach values of 15–20 times the annual average, while the minimum concentrations drop to one-twentieth of the annual average. The $SO_2$ concentrations increase slightly during the colder months, but they do not follow the pattern of smoke concentrations. This is probably so because local space heating (particularly wood burning) generates black smoke, but only minor quantities of $SO_2$.

A similar analysis for Auckland, New Zealand, shows a similar pattern, but with smoke concentrations almost an order of magnitude less than at Christchurch. Since the temperature in Auckland rarely drops below 10°C, space heating is much less frequent there.

## Variation of mean with maximum values

An additional analysis of the variability of pollutant data can be made by comparing the annual means of daily measurements with the 98th percentile values. This is illustrated by the scatter diagrams of $\bar{x}$ against $P_{98}$ in Fig. 16. The linear regression analyses of the points are summarized on each plot by the linear correlation coefficient $r$ and the coefficients A and B of the linear regression equation $P_{98} = A\bar{x} + B$. A fairly systematic relationship is seen between the mean and $P_{98}$ values, even though the data come from cities with fundamentally different meteorological, topographical, and socioeconomic characteristics. This relationship is different for $SO_2$, smoke, and SPM (high-volume) measurements. The high intercepts (B values) with the $P_{98}$ axis and the absence of combinations of low $\bar{x}$ and low $P_{98}$ values are to be noted, especially for SPM (high-volume) measurements. As pointed out in the $\sigma_g$ analysis, the $\bar{x} - P_{98}$ relationship confirms the smaller variability of the SPM (high-volume) measurements. This is not easily visually apparent in Fig. 18 because the $\bar{x}$ scale has been contracted in the plot of the SPM (high-volume) measurements.

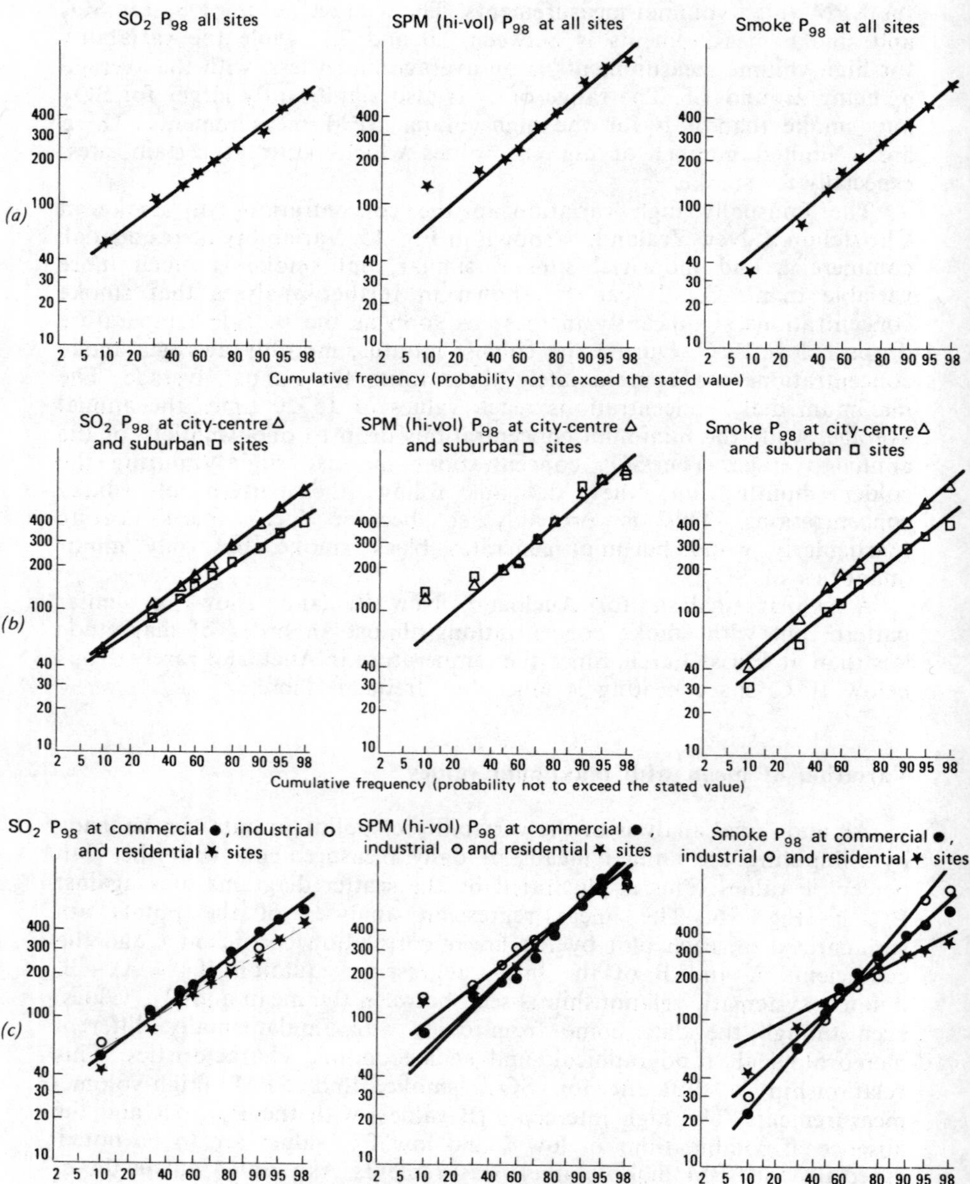


**Fig. 13. Cumulative frequency distributions of annual maximum values ($P_{98}$) of $SO_2$, SPM (gravimetric method), and smoke for 1973–1980 (*a*) at all sites, (*b*) at city-centre (CC), and suburban (S) sites, and (*c*) at commercial (C), industrial (I), and residential (R) sites**

## Comparison of SPM and smoke measurements made by different methods

Different methods are used for determining $SO_2$ and SPM concentrations at the various sites sampled in this project (see page 6). Thus, in order to overcome difficulties in interpreting data obtained by different methods, a comparison of methods is essential.

Simultaneous measurements of SPM concentrations by the two main methods (gravimetric and smoke-shade) have been carried out over several years at three sites in Tehran as well as at three sites in Copenhagen. Comparisons of results obtained by the nephelometer method and those obtained by the high-volume method have also been made at various sites, although on a much smaller scale compared with comparisons between results obtained by the high-volume and smoke-shade methods. The results of these comparisons are given in Table 3.

The ratios of SPM determinations by different methods are site dependent and also vary as a function of time at the same site. In the first entry, for example, for the commercial site in Copenhagen, the high-volume to smoke ratio of 1.9 is the average of the values 2, 2.5, 2, and 1.3 in successive years.

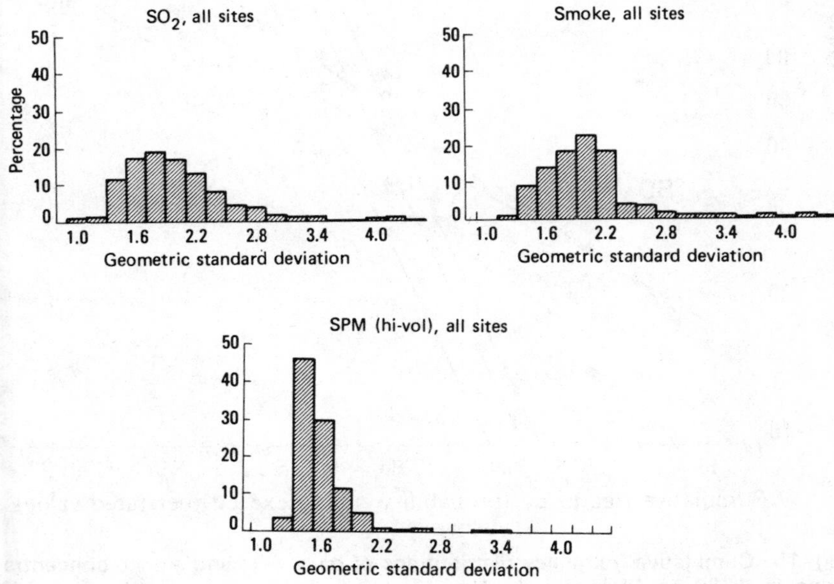


Fig. 14. Distribution of geometric standard deviations ($\sigma_g$) from the log-normal plots of daily average levels of $SO_2$, smoke, and SPM (high-volume) from all representative yearly data sets from all sites, 1973–1980

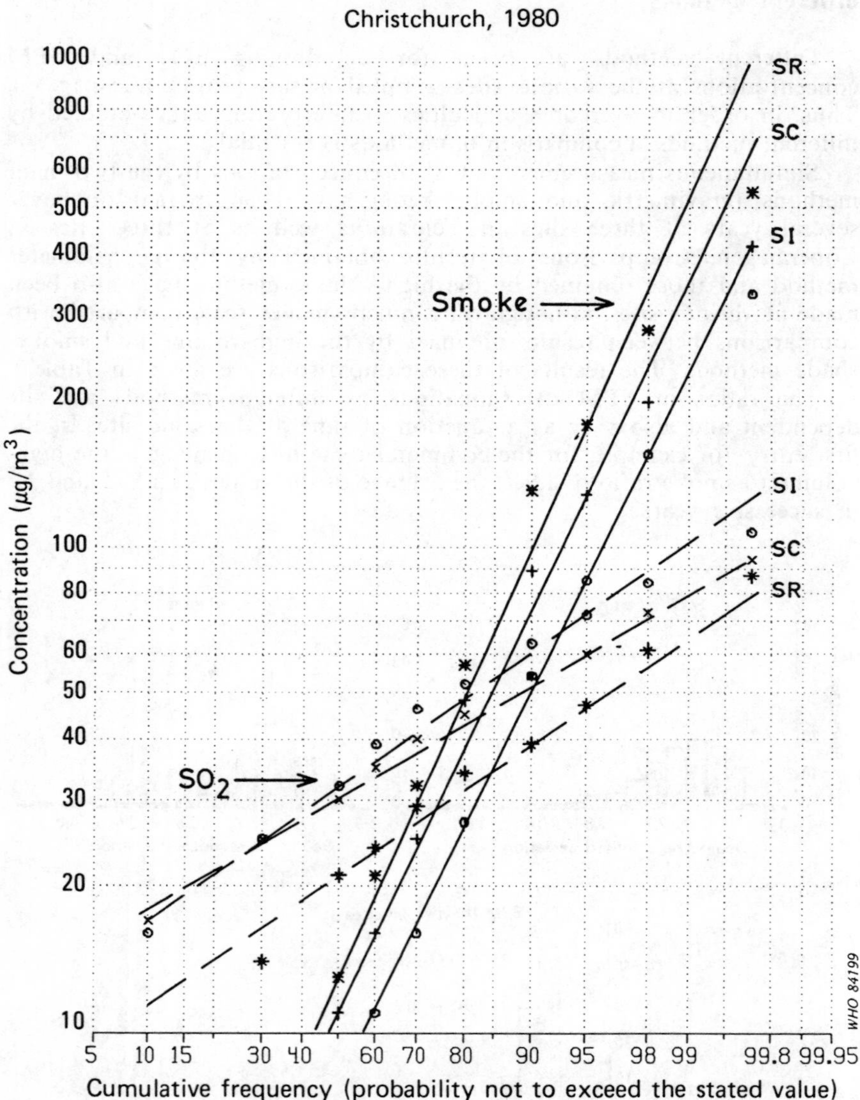


Fig. 15. Cumulative frequency distributions of daily $SO_2$ and smoke concentrations in 1980 at Christchurch, New Zealand, at suburban residential (SR), suburban commercial (SC), and suburban industrial (SI) sites

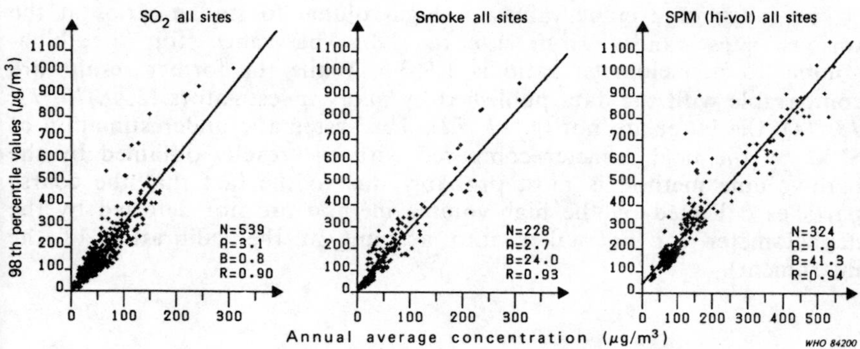


Fig. 16. Scatter diagrams of annual average ($\bar{x}$) and daily maximum ($P_{98}$) values for $SO_2$, smoke, and SPM (high-volume method) at all sites for 1973–1980

Table 3. Comparisons between methods for determining suspended particulate matter concentrations

| Site[a] | Period | No. of data | Concentrations (μg/m³) | | Ratio | Linear correlation coefficient |
|---|---|---|---|---|---|---|
| | | | *High-volume–smoke comparisons* | | | |
| Copenhagen | | | Hi-vol | Smoke | | |
| CCC | 1977–80 | 1 400 | 32 | 17 | 1.9 | 0.5–0.6 |
| SC | 1977–80 | 1 350 | 31 | 10 | 3.1 | 0.5–0.7 |
| SI | 1978–80 | 800 | 49 | 13 | 3.8 | 0.4 |
| Tehran | | | | | | |
| CCC | 1976–80 | 304 | 329 | 211 | 1.6 | 0–0.6 |
| SI | 1976–80 | 225 | 442 | 233 | 1.9 | 0–0.4 |
| SR | 1976–80 | 241 | 316 | 119 | 2.7 | 0–0.7 |
| | | | *High-volume-nephelometer comparisons* | | | |
| Manila | | | Hi-vol | Nephelometer | | |
| SI | 1978 | 36 | 246 | 71 | 3.5 | 0.8 |
| | 1979 | 49 | 279 | 86 | 3.2 | 0.4 |
| | 1980 | 31 | 122 | 83 | 1.5 | 0.2 |
| Melbourne | | | | | | |
| CCC | 1979 | 38 | 65 | 29 | 2.2 | 0.5 |
| Tokyo | | | | | | |
| CCI | 1978–79 | 33 | 140 | 67 | 2.1 | 0.6 |

[a] Site types: CCC, city-centre commercial; SC, suburban commercial; SI, suburban industrial; SR, suburban residential; CCI, city-centre industrial.

The range of average values of high-volume to smoke ratios at the various sites ranges from 1.6 to 3.8. The range for the high-volume to nephelometer ratio is 1.5–3.5. While the former results are comparable with the data published by many investigators (*2*, *9*, *10*, *11*, *13*, *14*), the latter are not (*4*, *11*, *12*). The systematic underestimation of SPM by the nephelometer compared with the results obtained by the high-volume method is most probably due to the fact that the coarse particles collected by the high-volume method are not detected by the nephelometer (or not taken into account in the calibration of the instrument).

# Correlation studies

In addition to a general view of the common variables of the data set, there are a number of correlations which may be made, specifically between results at the various sites within a city and between pollutants measured at the same site. The detailed interpretation of such correlations will be limited by the lack of information on the local source configuration and release patterns, and the meteorological conditions at the site.

A point to be made with regard to the outcome of correlations calculated from the GEMS air quality data from urban areas is the fundamental heterogeneity of the collected data. The term "urban area" covers a wide range of physical situations when applied on a global scale. The topography, spatial extent, and populations of urban areas differ markedly. Other factors affecting the measurements of pollutant concentrations include: local climatology; land-use zoning and housing; industrialization; and changing source configurations.

## Correlations between sites within a city

In considering the daily averages of air pollutant concentrations, it may be noted that the meteorological conditions affecting the transport, dispersion, and eventual removal of the pollutants from air are quite often the same for all measuring sites in an urban area, except in very specific topographic situations. While specific sources could highly influence the local concentrations at a specific site under well defined short-term meteorological conditions, the general meteorological features influence the variability at all sites in the same way. The former lowers the correlation between concentrations measured simultaneously at different sites in the same urban area and the latter increases it.

Highly variable relationships between the pollutant concentrations measured at different sites in the same urban area may be expected from the wide range of conditions in urban areas of the GEMS network. Fig. 17 illustrates the histograms of the linear correlation coefficients of $SO_2$, smoke, and gravimetrically determined SPM concentrations (high-

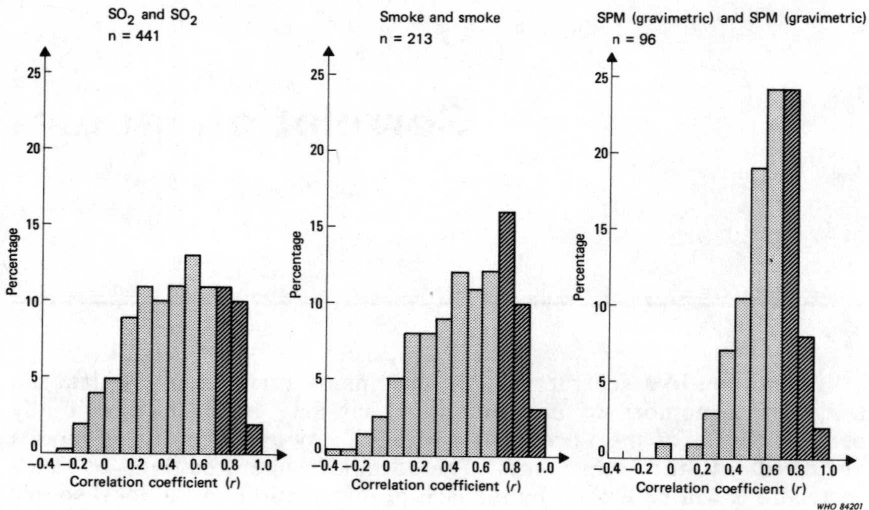


Fig. 17. Distribution of linear correlation coefficients for $SO_2$, smoke, and SPM (gravimetric) at two sites within the same urban area

volume and membrane samplers) measured at two sites within the same urban area. The linear correlation coefficients of yearly sets of paired daily averages in fact span a fairly wide range.

Annual data sets for which there were at least 40 simultaneously measured pairs of daily average values of pollutant concentrations were accepted for the correlation analysis. There were 441 such data sets for $SO_2$–$SO_2$ combinations and 213 for smoke–smoke combinations; of these, some 25% had at least 150 simultaneously measured pairs of daily average values, increasing the signficance level of the correlation. There were 96 SPM–SPM (gravimetric) combinations, many with more limited amounts of data (50–70 paired values each).

The distributions of correlation coefficients in Fig. 17 are similar for $SO_2$–$SO_2$ and smoke–smoke combinations, both being slightly skewed to the left. The SPM–SPM (gravimetric) distribution is more symmetric, centred on $r \simeq 0.6$. Very small correlation coefficient ($r$) values occurred frequently, especially for the $SO_2$–$SO_2$ and smoke–smoke combinations; in some cases even negative values were noted, though in general at very low levels of significance.

The shaded areas of the histograms in Fig. 17 represent the number of cases with a linear correlation coefficient of at least 0.7. These cases imply that at least 50% ($100r^2$) of the variability at one site can be associated with the variability at the other site in the urban area. The proportions in this category were 23% for $SO_2$–$SO_2$, 29% for smoke–smoke, and 34% for SPM–SPM (gravimetric) combinations.

It should be noted, however, that the higher correlations were not randomly distributed over the whole of the network. In fact, only a limited number of cities provided high correlations. For $SO_2$, 55 of 101 site combinations with $r \geqslant 0.7$ were from Zagreb (20), Amsterdam (14), Osaka (12), and Prague (9), with the remainder coming from 16 other cities. For smoke, the situation was similar, with 37 of 63 cases coming from Christchurch (9), Copenhagen (9), Auckland (8), London (6), and São Paulo (5), and the remainder from 11 other urban areas. For gravimetrically determined SPM concentrations, the situation was even simpler, with high correlations being given by the membrane sampler measurements in Zagreb (8) and the high-volume measurements in Birmingham (6), New York City (5), Toronto (5), Vancouver (4), St Louis (2), Montreal (1), and Pasadena (1).

It was investigated whether particular types of site were included in the cases of higher correlation, but all possible combinations of commercial, industrial, and residential sites were represented, with no predominance of any specific combination of site types.

Although detailed analyses of local situations are in general not within the scope of this report, it is of interest to give some examples of more in-depth treatment of selected data sets. Table 4 gives the results of correlations of $SO_2$ concentrations at the three GEMS sites in Amsterdam. Correlation increased quite steadily over the years for each possible combination of sites, possibly implying that intercomparability of the measurements had improved and that important local sources had been gradually eliminated. There were striking exceptions, however, for the combinations commercial–residential and commercial–industrial sites in 1974 and 1975. The sudden drop in correlation might have been due to various physical causes. An examination of the monthly and daily records of measurements showed the questionable or unusual periods in which the synchronism of variations was disturbed.

In Amsterdam and many other cities, the general seasonal meteorological pattern plays a very important role in the systematically high,

Table 4. Linear correlation[a] between daily $SO_2$ concentrations measured simultaneously at three different sites in Amsterdam: city-centre commercial (CCC), suburban residential (SR), and suburban industrial (SI)

| Year | CCC-SR | | CCC-SI | | SI-SR | |
|---|---|---|---|---|---|---|
| 1973 | 0.82 | (307) | 0.59 | (305) | 0.64 | (305) |
| 1974 | 0.64 | (342) | 0.42 | (333) | 0.66 | (333) |
| 1975 | 0.51 | (333) | 0.48 | (329) | 0.73 | (344) |
| 1976 | 0.88 | (340) | 0.81 | (335) | 0.78 | (335) |
| 1977 | 0.82 | (314) | 0.75 | (301) | 0.73 | (341) |
| 1978 | 0.89 | (279) | 0.89 | (269) | 0.85 | (298) |
| 1979 | 0.97 | (342) | 0.93 | (321) | 0.95 | (322) |

[a] Values given are the linear correlation coefficients, $r$. The figures in parentheses are the numbers of available simultaneous daily measurements.

positive correlations between the different sites. A regrouping of the data by season immediately lowers the correlation between sites; however, it gives a more objective measure of the relationship between simultaneously measured pollutant concentrations at different sites within the same urban area. Especially in studies aiming at the evaluation of the spatial representativeness of a limited number of monitoring sites for a larger area, the influence of seasonal cycles must be determined and eliminated before starting the analysis, as has been pointed out, for example, in some studies carried out in New York City (*7, 8*). In the above-mentioned cities (page 35), where high correlations between sites were noted, seasonal cycles always played a major role.

Another example of a more detailed correlation analysis is given in Fig. 18 for the SPM (high-volume) measurements in Toronto during 1978–1980. A discontinuous sampling scheme is used, providing around 50 paired values each year. The scatter diagrams show how markedly the patterns change from year to year. A high correlation was seen between SPM at the commercial and industrial site in 1979, but correlations were not as high in 1978 and 1980.

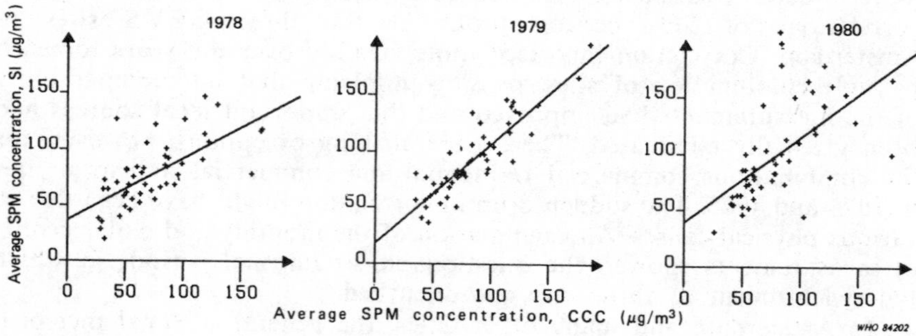


**Fig. 18. Scatter diagrams of SPM (high-volume) simultaneous measurements at the suburban industrial (SI) and city-centre commercial (CCC) sites in Toronto in 1978, 1979, and 1980**

A final example of correlation between simultaneous measurements of pollutant concentrations is given in Table 5 for the three GEMS sites in London. There are changing numbers of simultaneous measurements from year to year, and thus a variable correlation pattern. The sudden complete lack of correlation, in 1977, between the industrial site and the other two sites is, however, quite striking. An examination of the data sets shows that, during March 1977, the smoke concentrations at the industrial site were about 5 times higher than those recorded at the other two sites; normally, the concentrations at all sites are similar. Data are missing for the industrial site from June to November 1977, which supports the assumption that something abnormal happened at this

Table 5. Linear correlation[a] between daily smoke concentrations measured simultaneously at three different sites in London: city-centre commercial (CCC), suburban residential (SR), and suburban industrial (SI)

| Year | CCC-SR | | CCC-SI | | SI-SR | |
|---|---|---|---|---|---|---|
| 1973 | 0.74 | (125) | 0.77 | (122) | 0.80 | (110) |
| 1974 | 0.71 | (200) | 0.68 | (162) | 0.76 | (151) |
| 1975 | 0.88 | (193) | 0.47 | (164) | 0.46 | (154) |
| 1976 | 0.59 | (199) | 0.41 | (139) | 0.68 | (130) |
| 1977 | 0.68 | (206) | 0.10 | (139) | 0.01 | ( 78) |
| 1978 | 0.51 | (297) | 0.45 | (335) | 0.48 | (267) |

[a] Values given are the linear correlation coefficient, *r*. The figures in parentheses are the numbers of available simultaneous daily measurements.

particular site in March 1977, and that the reported smoke data may not at all be representative for that year. This example clearly illustrates the usefulness of correlation techniques (when applied correctly) in drawing attention to abnormal or unusual phenomena occurring during limited periods in the area of the monitoring site.

On the basis of the studies of linear correlations between the concentrations of the same pollutant measured simultaneously at different sites within an urban area, it can be stated that:

— As expected on the basis of the very different local conditions in the various urban areas supplying data to the GEMS air data bank, correlations between sites for a given pollutant are quite different from one city to another and a wide range of values is observed.

— For each of the pollutants under investigation, the correlations between sites are generally significant, although the median values of the linear correlation coefficients do not exceed 0.6.

— In certain cities, there is a marked and persistent incidence of high or of low correlations, with few exceptions from one year to another. In other cities or for other combinations of sites within a city, correlations vary in an almost random way from one year to another. The reasons for this can only be determined by means of a detailed analysis, taking into account additional information, most of which is available only at the local level. These phenomena certainly deserve further attention in any subsequent monitoring activities.

— Seasonal cycles in the local air pollution levels influence correlations between different sites. Any more detailed study attempting to reveal relationships between sites other than those governed by local meteorology must first determine and eliminate this over-riding effect.

— Within a given city, the correlation between sites in a residential and a commercial area is not necessarily higher than the correlations between sites at industrial and residential, and industrial and commercial areas. This could indicate that, in general, sites in industrial areas are not under the direct influence of specific large sources of industrial pollution or, at any rate, that their impact is averaged out due to the fluctuations in wind direction within the 24-hour period used as the averaging time for the measurements.

## Correlations between pollutants at the same site

Correlations between $SO_2$ and SPM (determined gravimetrically or as smoke) have been investigated in the data available from the air monitoring project. As in the previous correlations, data sets were required to include at least 40 simultaneous determinations during the year. The distributions of the linear correlation coefficients are given in Fig. 19. The $SO_2$–smoke correlations benefited from larger data sets; 80% had more than 150 paired daily results, while only 20% of the $SO_2$–gravimetric SPM combinations had that many paired daily results. The difference is due to the more frequent discontinuous sampling schemes for SPM, especially with the high-volume method, e.g., one measurement every six days. Smoke determinations are made more continuously.

The histograms of linear correlation coefficients in Fig. 19 show the distributions of linear correlation coefficients between $SO_2$ and smoke and between $SO_2$ and gravimetric SPM determinations. The distribution of the $SO_2$ and smoke correlations is skewed to the left, with some 20% of the available correlations having linear correlation factors greater than

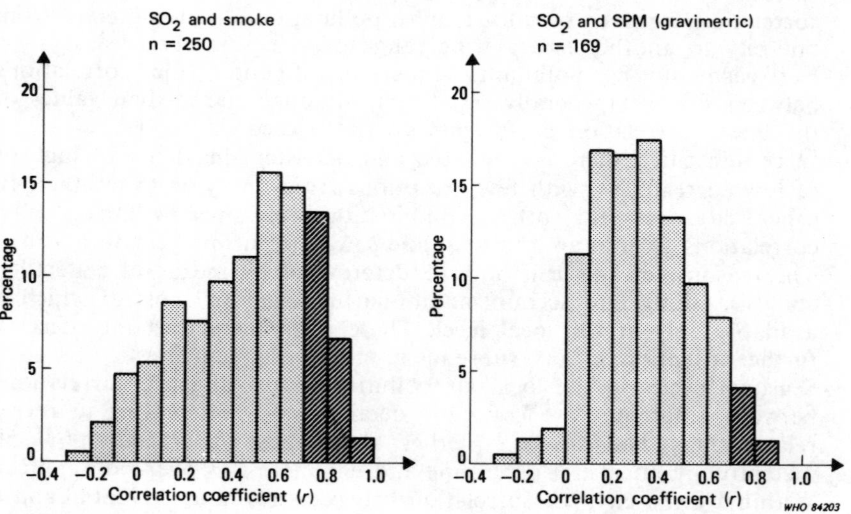


Fig. 19. Distributions of linear correlation coefficients between $SO_2$ and smoke and between $SO_2$ and SPM (gravimetric) measured simultaneously at individual sites throughout the network

0.7. The higher correlations were from 13 cities, but over half came from 4 cities: Brussels, Madrid, Santiago, and São Paulo.

The distribution of $SO_2$ and gravimetric SPM correlations is skewed to the right, with a median value of the linear correlation factors of not larger than 0.3. Less than 5% of these correlations have $r \geqslant 0.7$. The higher correlations come from Zagreb (4), Vancouver (1), Frankfurt (1), Calcutta (1), and St Louis (1).

When the $SO_2$ and smoke correlations were analysed with respect to site, the highest correlations were seen to occur at the sites in commercial areas, followed by sites in residential and industrial areas; in the case of industrial sites the correlations were very low.

As was the case for correlations between sites, the correlations between measurements at the same site are very sensitive to seasonal cycles. Synchronous temporal cycles in the concentrations of different pollutants measured at the same site increase the correlation between paired values. Care must, therefore, be taken to determine and eliminate this effect before trying to find any other (remaining) physical reasons for the observed correlations.

Although year to year variations in the degree of correlation between pollutants measured at the same site can occur under normal conditions, unusually abrupt changes deserve special attention, more particularly from the point of view of possible failures in sampling, analysis, or data treatment procedures.

# Comparisons with exposure limits published by WHO

The impact on human health of the air pollutant concentrations measured in the WHO/UNEP air monitoring project may be assessed by comparing the data with the WHO guidelines for exposure limits for $SO_2$, smoke, and SPM (Table 6). However, it should be pointed out at the outset that exposure (and hence the health risk) of individuals is difficult to estimate because of their movements through various zones (indoors and outdoors) of different air quality.

In 1979, WHO published exposure limits for $SO_2$ and suspended particulate matter, measured as smoke or determined gravimetrically, to limit the effects of both acute and long-term exposures (Table 6) (*19*). For long-term exposures and the related risks to public health, reference is made to the annual average pollutant concentrations in air. For short-term exposures and risks, the guideline applies to the 98th percentile value of the annual record of daily average concentrations.

Table 6. WHO Guidelines for exposure limits for $SO_2$, smoke and gravimetrically determined SPM consistent with the protection of public health

| | $SO_2$ ($\mu g/m^3$) | SPM ($\mu g/m^3$) | |
|---|---|---|---|
| | | Smoke | Gravimetric determination[a] |
| Yearly arithmetic average | 40–60 | 40–60 | 60–90 |
| 98th percentile of the daily averages | 100–150 | 100–150 | 150–230 |

[a] These figures are estimates intended to relate to high-volume sampler observations.

*Source*: reference *19*.

## Long-term exposure limits

In order to obtain representative annual average concentrations at each site of the network and to compare these values with the long-term exposure limits suggested by WHO, mean values were taken from the measurement period 1975–1980 from all sites; the results of the comparisons are given in Table 7.

With respect to the average $SO_2$ concentrations, nearly half of all sites are below the lower exposure limit published by WHO (40 $\mu g/m^3$), while one-quarter are above the upper limit (60 $\mu g/m^3$). Comparisons by type of site show that the limit values for $SO_2$ are more frequently exceeded at the city-centre sites compared with the suburban ones, and at the commercial and industrial sites compared with the residential ones. The data show that 60% of the residential sites have annual average $SO_2$ concentrations below the lower WHO limit.

With respect to SPM, somewhat more sites are above the upper limit compared with $SO_2$. Of all sites, just over 40% are above the upper SPM limit and a quarter are below the lower value. The pattern is similar for the breakdown between city-centre and suburban sites. A comparison of commercial, industrial, and residential sites shows that fewer industrial sites are below the lower limit and fewer residential sites are above the upper limit. The upper limit for annual average SPM is exceeded at half of the industrial sites. Although about 40% of the commercial sites exceed the SPM limit and a similar fraction exceed the $SO_2$ limit, only around 20% of all commercial sites simultaneously exceed both limits.

Table 7. Comparisons of GEMS network data with WHO exposure limits; percentage of sites with respect to guideline values

| Site | $SO_2$ | | | SPM | | |
|---|---|---|---|---|---|---|
| | Below | Within | Above | Below | Within | Above |
| | | | *Annual average (1975–1980)* | | | |
| All sites | 49 | 25 | 26 | 24 | 34 | 42 |
| City-centre | 41 | 28 | 31 | 23 | 33 | 44 |
| Suburban | 58 | 21 | 21 | 25 | 34 | 41 |
| Commercial | 37 | 26 | 37 | 26 | 30 | 44 |
| Industrial | 48 | 26 | 26 | 18 | 31 | 51 |
| Residential | 60 | 22 | 18 | 27 | 40 | 33 |
| | | | *98th percentile values (1978)* | | | |
| All sites | 43 | 24 | 32 | 30 | 23 | 47 |
| City-centre | 35 | 27 | 38 | 27 | 19 | 54 |
| Suburban | 53 | 21 | 26 | 34 | 27 | 39 |
| Commercial | 33 | 31 | 36 | 29 | 24 | 47 |
| Industrial | 47 | 14 | 39 | 29 | 18 | 53 |
| Residential | 51 | 29 | 20 | 32 | 26 | 42 |

# Trends

An important objective of the GEMS air monitoring network is to observe trends in the quality of urban air. Given the variability in pollutant concentrations in air, the time period for analysis (around 5–8 years) is short. In addition, the composition of the network has changed each year, mainly through the inclusion of additional sites; it is, therefore, not easy to observe overall trends in air pollution variables for the project. The trends at individual sites have, thus, been determined.

**Broad-based trends**

Trend analysis for the annual average $SO_2$ and SPM concentrations, and the $P_{98}$ values, was performed for each site having at least five successive years of representative data. This involved 63 sites; however, almost half of them had only 5 years of information available. For this reason, only a semi-quantitative procedure was used, namely the determination of the percentage change in the average results in the second half of the period compared with the average in the first half of the period. If there were odd numbers of years in the period available, the middle year was used in both halves. The result is expressed as the percentage change per year.

With this technique, judgement of the statistical significance of the trends is rather arbitrary. For classification purposes, a trend was said to be downward if the change was at least $-3\%$ per year and upward if the change was at least $+3\%$ per year.

The results of the trend analysis for changes in the annual average concentrations are given in Table 8, and for the 98th percentile values in Table 9. More details regarding the magnitude of the changes in these variables are given in Fig. 22 and 23.

The predominant trend in the $SO_2$ data is downward. In approximately 50% of the sites, the annual average concentrations and the $P_{98}$ values are decreasing. This observation is almost independent of the type of site, except in the case of sites in commercial areas, where up to 60% of the sites show downward trends. Upward trends are noted in

Table 8. Trends in annual averages of air pollutants, 1973–1980

| Site | No. of sites | Percentage of sites showing different trends | | |
|---|---|---|---|---|
| | | Downward | Stationary | Upward |
| *Sulfur dioxide* | | | | |
| All sites | 63 | 54 | 30 | 16 |
| City-centre | 34 | 56 | 26 | 18 |
| Suburban | 29 | 52 | 34 | 14 |
| Commercial | 23 | 61 | 17 | 22 |
| Industrial | 20 | 55 | 30 | 15 |
| Residential | 20 | 45 | 45 | 10 |
| *Suspended particulate matter* | | | | |
| All sites | 62 | 43 | 47 | 10 |
| City-centre | 34 | 47 | 47 | 6 |
| Suburban | 28 | 39 | 46 | 15 |
| Commercial | 21 | 38 | 52 | 10 |
| Industrial | 20 | 50 | 40 | 10 |
| Residential | 21 | 42 | 48 | 10 |

Table 9. Trends in 98th percentiles of air pollutants, 1973–1980

| Site | No. of sites | Percentage of sites showing different trends | | |
|---|---|---|---|---|
| | | Downward | Stationary | Upward |
| *Sulfur dioxide* | | | | |
| All sites | 62 | 50 | 23 | 27 |
| City-centre | 33 | 45 | 30 | 25 |
| Suburban | 29 | 55 | 14 | 31 |
| Commercial | 23 | 48 | 30 | 22 |
| Industrial | 19 | 53 | 21 | 26 |
| Residential | 20 | 50 | 15 | 35 |
| *Suspended particulate matter* | | | | |
| All sites | 61 | 43 | 36 | 21 |
| City-centre | 33 | 42 | 33 | 25 |
| Suburban | 28 | 43 | 39 | 18 |
| Commercial | 21 | 43 | 33 | 24 |
| Industrial | 19 | 53 | 16 | 31 |
| Residential | 21 | 33 | 57 | 10 |

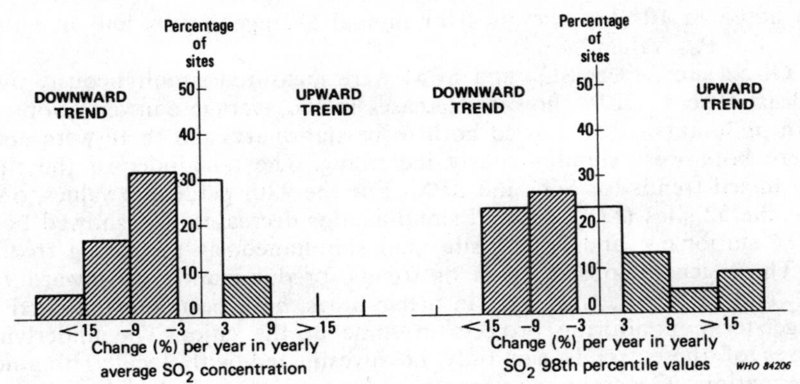


Fig. 22. Distribution of trends in annual average ($\bar{x}$) and daily maximum ($P_{98}$) values of $SO_2$ at all sites having at least five consecutive years of representative data

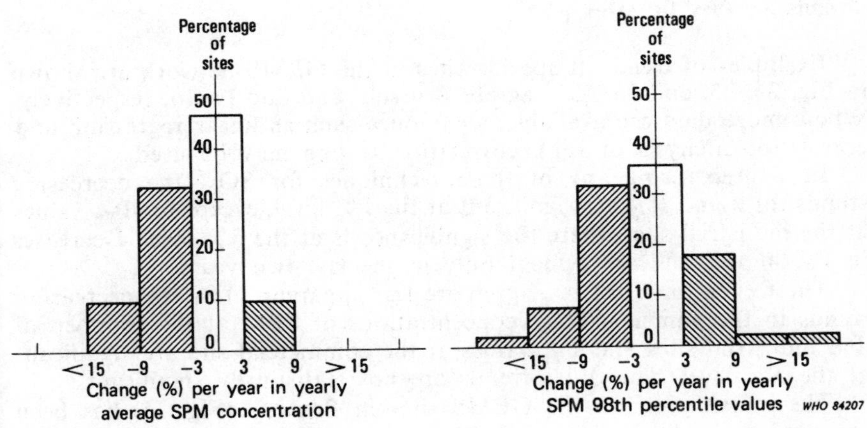


Fig. 23. Distribution of trends in annual average ($\bar{x}$) and daily maximum (P98) values of suspended particulate matter at all sites having at least five consecutive years of representative data

about 15% of the sites for annual average concentrations and 25% for the $P_{98}$ values. Most of the changes are in the range 3–9% per year, with fewer ranging from 9% to 15% per year or greater than 15% per year (Fig. 22).

The trends for SPM are also predominantly downward. Approximately 45% of the sites have decreasing annual average concentrations and $P_{98}$ values. A somewhat larger percentage of the industrial sites show downward trends, 50% or slightly more for both annual average concentrations and $P_{98}$ values. Upward trends in SPM are noted in 10% of the sites for annual average results and in about 20% for $P_{98}$ values.

Of 52 sites where $SO_2$ and SPM were measured simultaneously over at least 5 years, 30% showed decreases in the average concentrations of both pollutants, 20% showed both to be stationary, and there were none where both were simultaneously increasing. The remainder of the sites had mixed trends for $SO_2$ and SPM. For the 98th percentile values, only 9 of the 52 sites (17%) showed simultaneous decreases, 8% showed both to be stationary, and 2% (1 site) had simultaneously increasing trends.

These general observations of trends, predominantly downward for $SO_2$ and SPM concentrations in urban areas, have been substantiated in longer-term monitoring projects in some of the cities. The underlying causes of these trends can only be investigated with locally obtained information. Generally, lower air pollutant concentrations are attributable to emission reduction systems, the use of low-sulfur fuels, energy conservation policies, and higher stacks to increase dispersion.

## Trends at specific sites

Examples of trends at specific sites in the GEMS network are shown in Fig. 24, 25, and 26, for Zagreb, Brussels, and São Paulo, respectively. Where more data are available, techniques such as linear regression and correlation analysis or rank correlation testing may be used.

In Zagreb, using any of these techniques for $SO_2$, the decreasing trends for $\bar{x}$ and $P_{98}$ are significant at the 1% level, except for $P_{98}$ values at the industrial site, where the significance is at the 5% level. Decreases in $P_{98}$ at this site are evident only in the last two years.

The trends for SPM in Zagreb are less apparent. Only the decreasing trends in the annual average concentrations of SPM at the commercial and industrial sites and $P_{98}$ values at the commercial site are significant at the 5% level. The other trends are not statistically significant.

The information on the GEMS sites in Brussels (Fig. 25) has been extended over the period 1969–1981 with additional monitoring data. Linear regression analysis on these data reveals highly significant (1% level) downward trends. If the GEMS data alone, for the limited period 1973–1980, are considered at these sites, there are less pronounced decreases and therefore the trends are statistically less significant.

The trends in air pollutant concentrations in São Paulo, illustrated in Fig. 26, are more complicated to interpret. Each of the three sites is designated city-centre. Annual average concentrations and 98th percentile smoke values decreased during the five years 1976–1980 at all sites, with decreases ranging from 5% to 11% per year. The concentrations of $SO_2$, on the other hand, were stationary at the industrial site, but increased by 5–10% per year at the commercial and residential sites. Information at the local level (*6*) indicates that attention has been focused on reducing highly visible black smoke rather than on reducing $SO_2$ emissions.

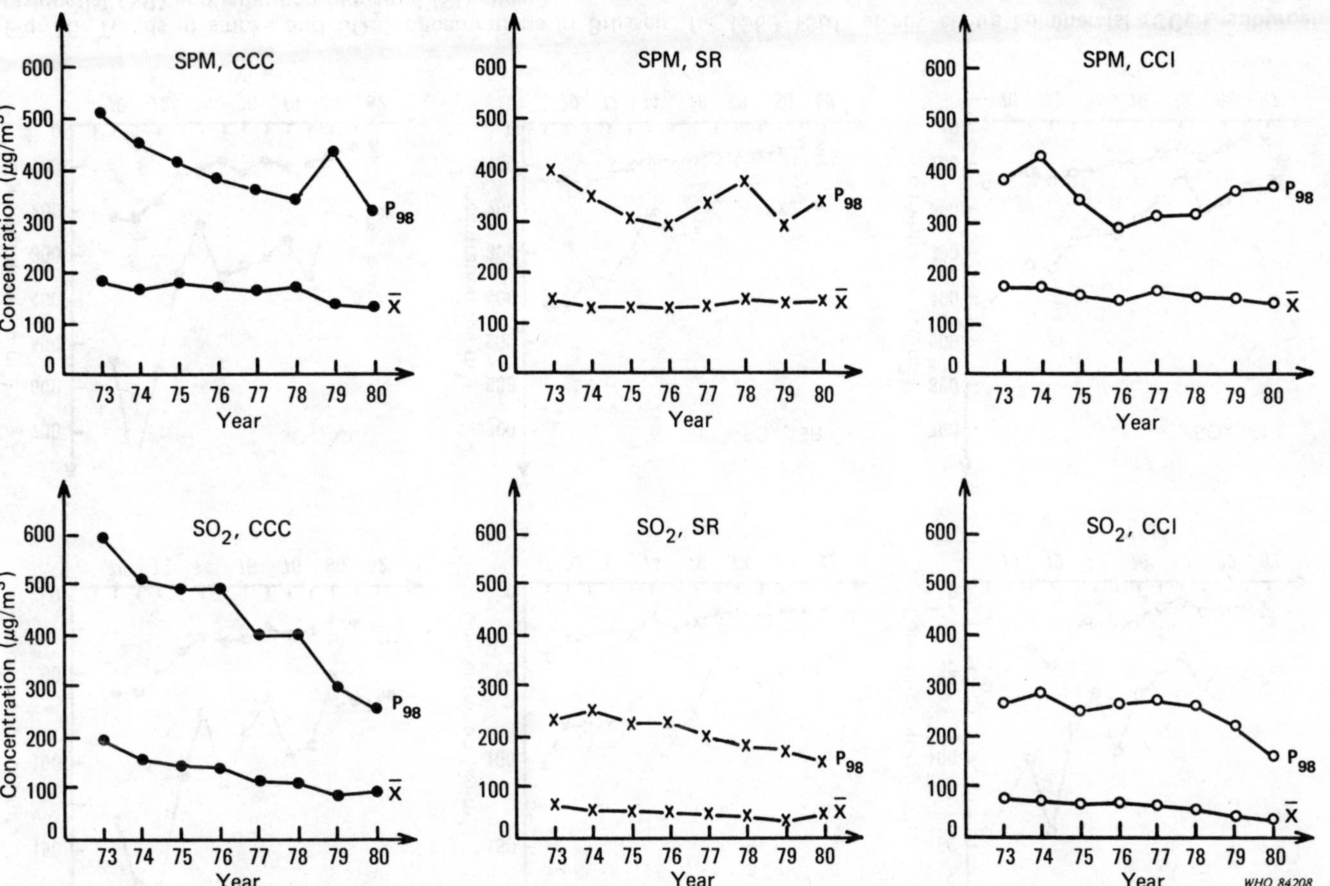


Fig. 24. Trends in SPM and $SO_2$ concentrations in Zagreb, for 1973–1980, at city-centre commercial (CCC), suburban residential (SR) and city-centre industrial (CCI) sites

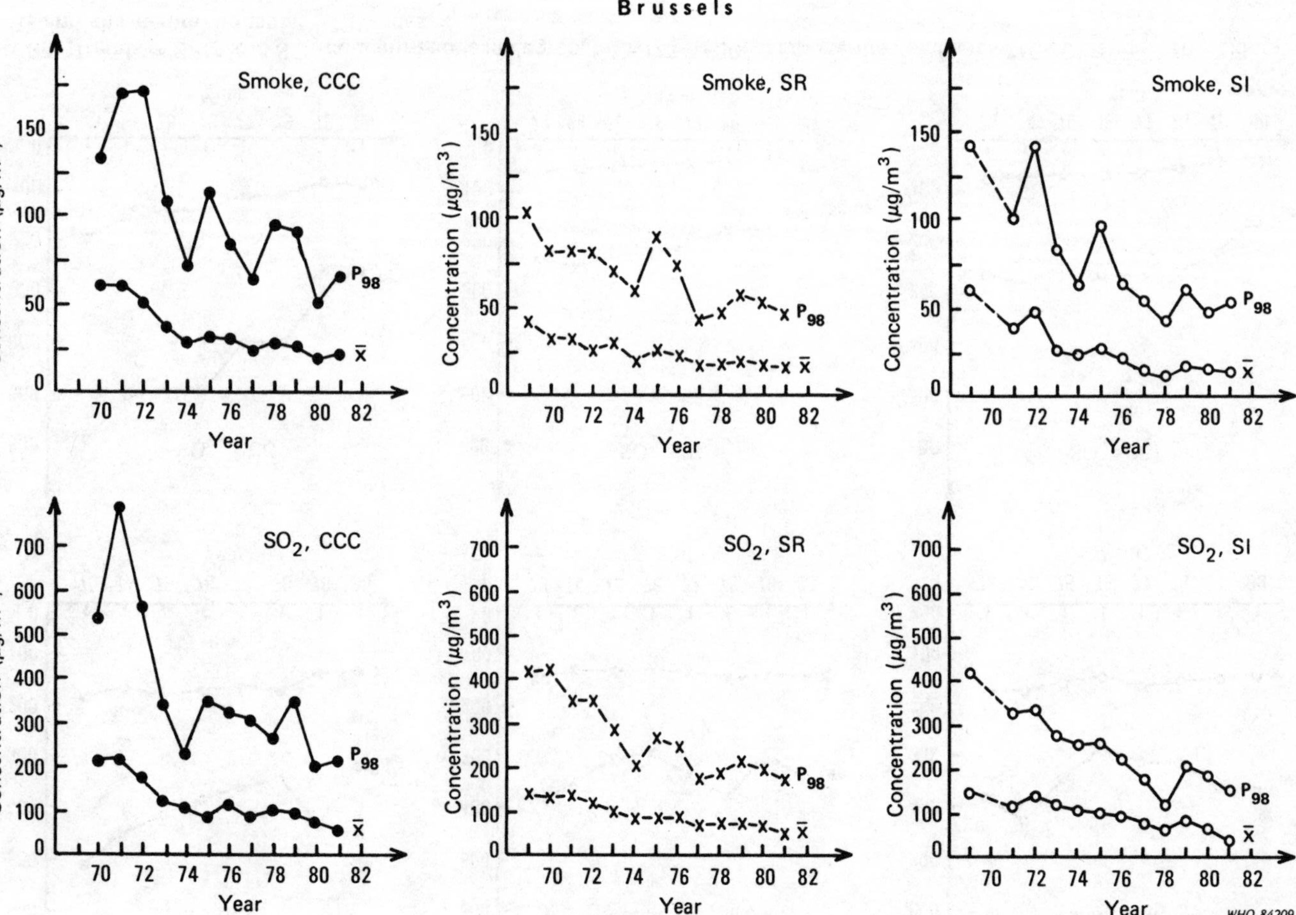


Fig. 25. Trends in smoke and $SO_2$ concentrations in Brussels, for 1969–1981, at city-centre commercial (CCC), suburban residential (SR) and suburban industrial (SI) sites

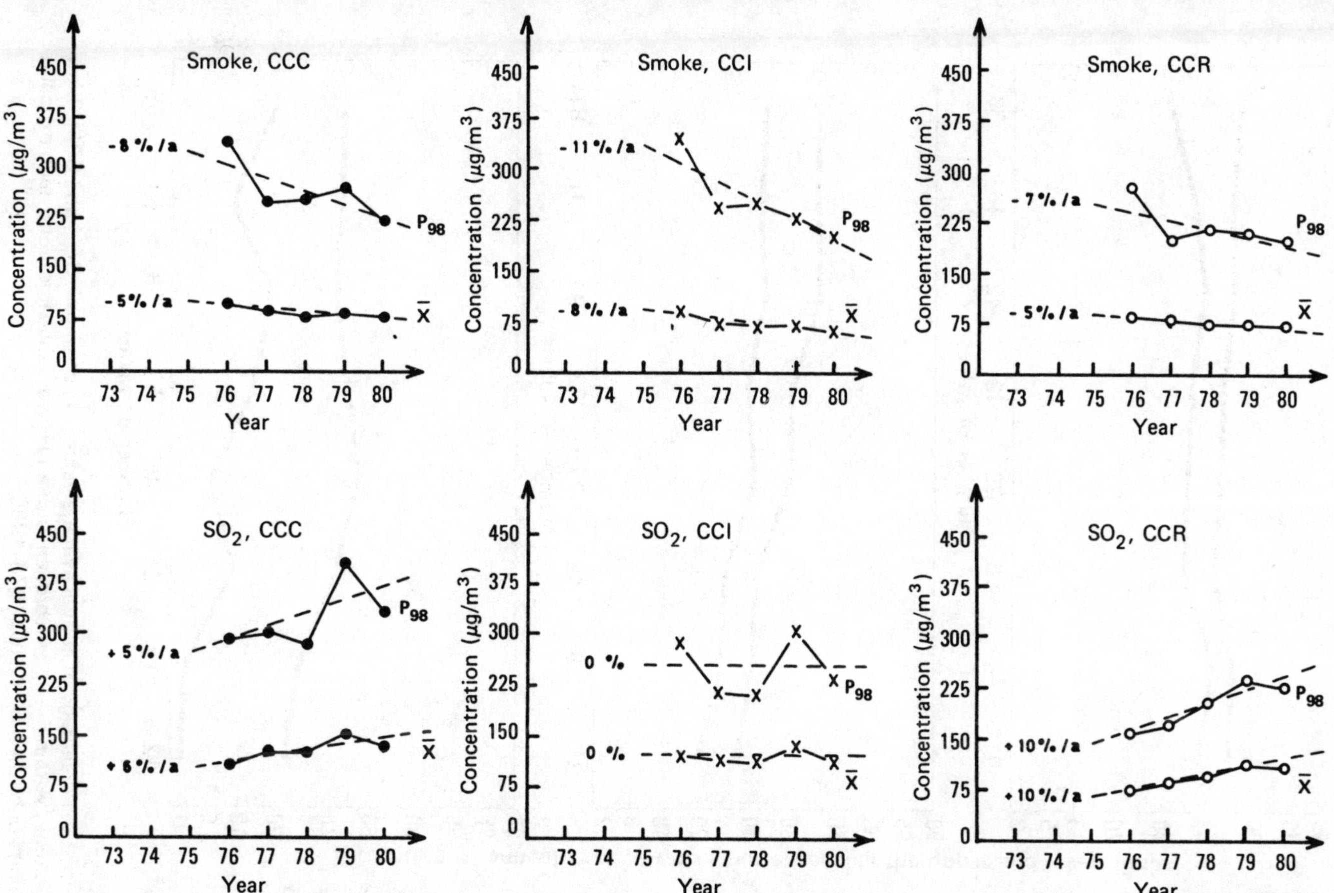


Fig. 26. Trends in smoke and $SO_2$ concentrations in São Paulo, for 1976–1980, at city-centre commercial (CCC), city-centre industrial (CCI) and city-centre residential (CCR) sites

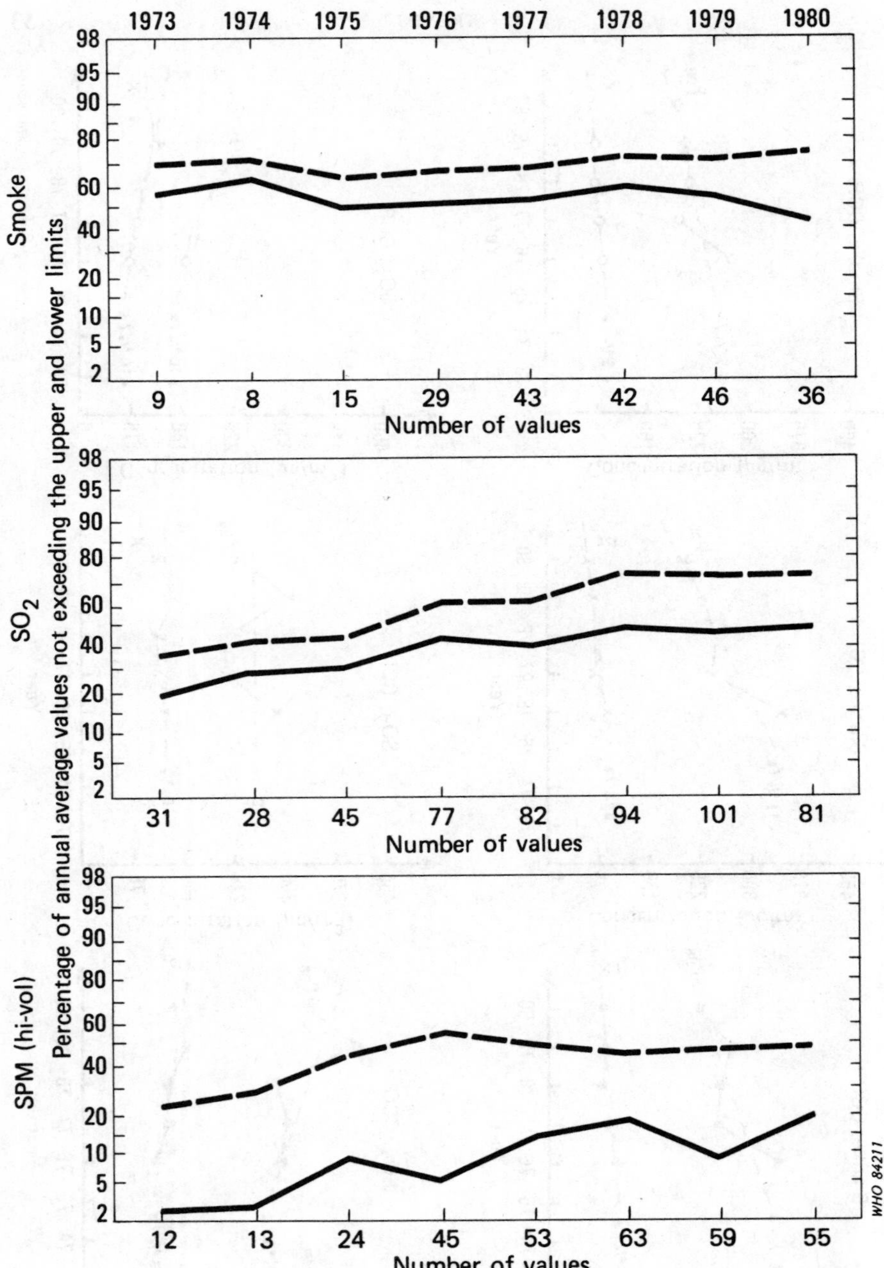


Fig. 27. Percentage of annual average values ($\bar{x}$) of smoke, $SO_2$, and SPM (high-volume) within the upper (broken line) and lower (solid line) long-term exposure limits published by WHO, 1973–1980

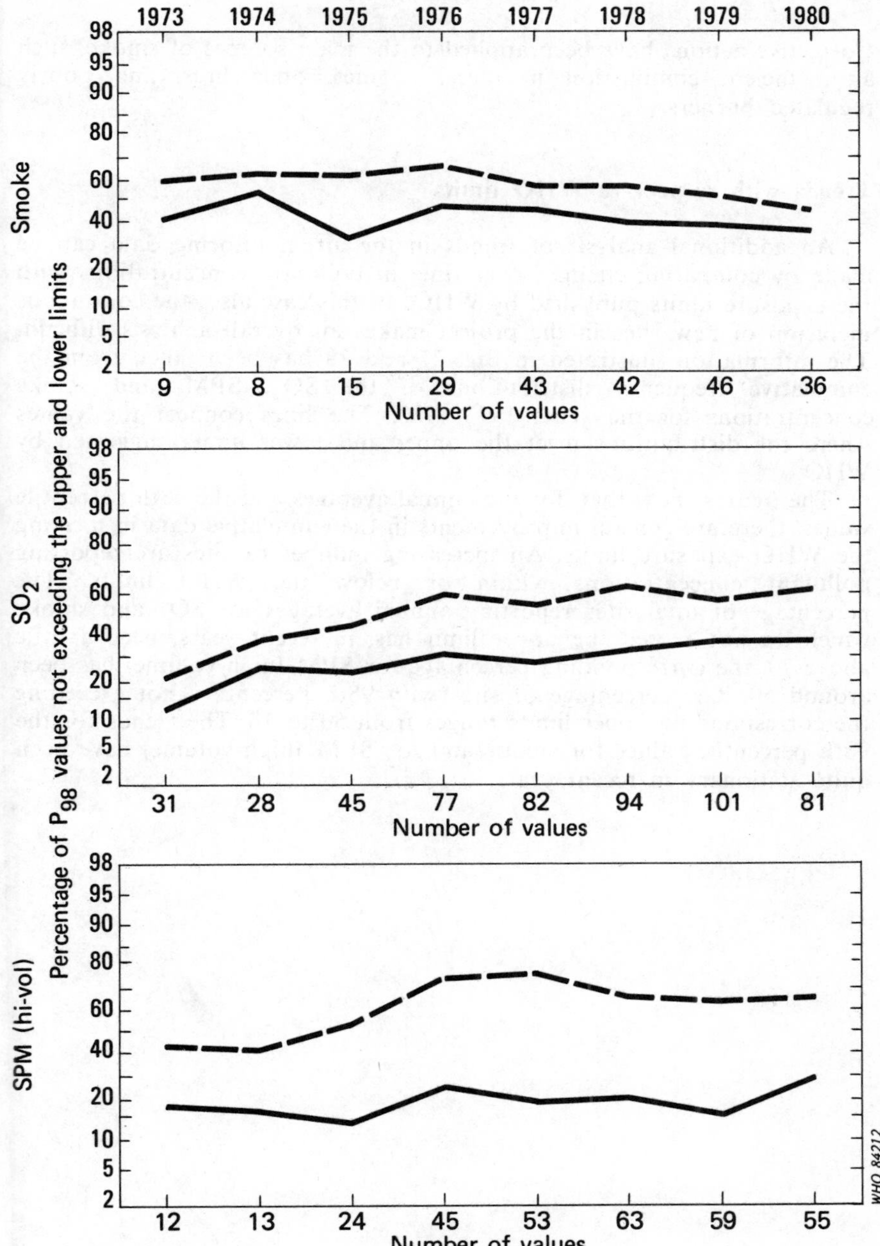


Fig. 28. Percentage of $P_{98}$ values of smoke, $SO_2$, and SPM (high-volume) within the upper (broken line) and lower (solid line) short-term exposure limits published by WHO, 1973–1980

Corrective actions have been applied to the main sources of smoke, such as inefficient combustion in diesel engines, open fires, and poorly regulated burners.

## Trends with respect to WHO limits

An additional analysis of trends in the air monitoring data can be made by comparing changes over time in pollutant concentrations with the exposure limits published by WHO. In this case also, the continuous inclusion of new sites in the project makes an overall analysis difficult. The information illustrated in Fig. 27 and 28 has been taken from the cumulative frequency distributions of the $SO_2$, SPM, and smoke concentrations for the years 1973–1980. The lines connect the values where the distributions meet the upper and lower limits suggested by WHO.

The figures show that, for the annual averages and the 98th percentile values, there are general improvements in the cumulative data in meeting the WHO exposure limits. An increasing number of sites are reporting pollutant concentrations within or below the WHO limits. The percentage of total sites reporting annual averages for $SO_2$ and smoke which do not exceed the upper limit has, in recent years, been a little above 70; the corresponding percentage for SPM (high-volume) has been around 50. The percentage of sites with 98th percentiles not exceeding the corresponding upper limits ranges from 50 to 70. The trends for the 98th percentile values for smoke and for SPM (high-volume) have been quite stationary in recent years.

# Summary and conclusions

The WHO/UNEP global air monitoring project has developed considerably since its inception in 1973. The network has expanded to include sites in about 70 cities in some 35 countries. There are sufficient sites in the network to give a broad, global view of urban air pollution, although important geographical areas lack coverage, particularly Central America, Africa, and the USSR.

Approximately 60 000 daily average values of $SO_2$ and suspended particulate matter are recorded in the data bank each year. For the most part, measurements at each site are distributed sufficiently evenly throughout the year to give representative annual averages. It is generally satisfactory to report the cumulative frequency distributions of daily measurements and the annual average results, as is done in biennial reports of the project (*17*, *18*, *20*, *22*). This is the first interpretative analysis of the data obtained in the period 1973–1980.

As can be expected from the wide diversity of sites, local conditions, and pollution sources, there are wide ranges in measurement results. For the data as a whole, the median annual average concentrations were 44 $\mu g/m^3$ for $SO_2$, 35 $\mu g/m^3$ for smoke, and 85 $\mu g/m^3$ for suspended particulate matter (high-volume results). Generally, lower levels of pollution were recorded at suburban and residential sites than at city-centre, commercial, and industrial sites.

The relationships of results within individual urban areas have been investigated in correlation analyses. For cities with two or three sites, a high correlation ($r > 0.7$) was found for the $SO_2$ data in one-quarter of the sites and for the SPM data in about a third of the sites. Correlations between the concentrations of $SO_2$ and suspended particulate matter, measured at the same site, were also made. The correlations varied quite widely, with seasonal cycles exerting a strong influence. Such correlations are particularly useful in drawing attention to unusual environmental conditions or to abnormal monitoring operations.

In most urban areas the pollutant concentrations were within or below the exposure limits suggested by WHO for the protection of human health. About 25–30% of the sites reported annual averages and maximum daily concentrations of $SO_2$ above the upper limit value and around 40–50% of the sites did so for the concentrations of suspended particulate matter. The specific exposure of individuals is not known because of the undetermined movement of individuals through temporally and spatially varying air quality conditions.

An important objective of the GEMS network is to observe the time trends in urban air pollution. The time period for monitoring results of the network is still relatively short, but trends were determined for 63 sites for which at least 5 years' information was available. The predominant trend in air pollution levels at these sites was downward. Upward trends were noted in the annual average at 10 sites for $SO_2$ and 6 sites for suspended particulate matter concentrations (greater than 3% per year change between the first and second halves of the monitoring period). Of 52 sites at which both $SO_2$ and suspended particulate matter were measured, there were none with simultaneously increasing trends.

The cities in which increasing trends in air pollution were noted have not been specifically identified. It is to be expected, however, that these are areas of increasing population growth and industrial development. Many sites included in the trend analysis had data only for the past 5 years. The continuation of the monitoring project should, of course, provide more definitive results.

The GEMS quality assurance programme has been directed towards: (*a*) monitoring system design and operator training; (*b*) method performance and inter-method comparison studies; and (*c*) data validation. In the first area, guideline documents have been produced which discuss monitoring methods, network design, and data analysis and interpretation (*15*, *16*, *21*). Training has also been provided as required. In the second area, audits of $SO_2$ have been carried out using standard reference materials. In addition, comparison studies of the methods of measuring $SO_2$ and SPM concentrations have taken place at several locations throughout the network. In the latter area, data validation checks are being incorporated into the data management system to provide better quality data for data assessment and interpretation.

The data accumulated through the air monitoring project show the broad features of urban air pollution. As such, they provide a global picture of urban air quality. This is a useful perspective for the more specific interpretation of locally obtained monitoring results, which requires additional information on local emission sources and environmental conditions. The use of specific local information to explain or interpret globally observed features has been illustrated in the text.

# References

1. APLING, A. J. ET AL. *The high pollution episode in London, December 1975.* Stevenage, Warren Spring Laboratory, 1977 (LR 263 (AP)).
2. BALL, D. J. & HUME, R. The relative importance of vehicular and domestic emissions of dark smoke in Greater London in the mid-1970s. *Atmospheric environment*, **11**: 1065–1073 (1977).
3. CEC. *Exchange of information concerning atmospheric pollution by certain sulphur compounds and suspended particulates in the European Community.* Annual Report for January to December 1977. Luxembourg, Commission for the European Communities, 1980 (EUR 6827 EN).
4. CHARLSON, R. J. ET AL. On the generality of correlation of atmospheric aerosol mass concentration and light scatter. *Atmospheric environment*, **2**: 455–464 (1968).
5. DE KONING, H. & KÖHLER, A. Monitoring global air pollution. *Environmental science and technology*, **12**: 884–889 (1978).
6. DERISIO, J. C. & ONISHI, E. Y. The air pollution control and the corrective action in the greater São Paulo area. In: *Proceedings of the 5th International Clean Air Congress, Argentina, 1982.* pp. 1024–1028.
7. GOLDSTEIN, I. F. ET AL. Air pollution patterns in New York City. *Journal of the Air Pollution Control Association*, **24**: 148–152 (1974).
8. GOLDSTEIN, I. F. & LANDOVITZ, L. Analysis of air pollution patterns in New York City – Can one aerometric station represent the area surrounding it? *Atmospheric environment*, **11**: 47–57 (1977).
9. GRIGGS, M. Relationship of optical observations to aerosol mass loading. *Journal of the Air Pollution Control Association*, **22**: 148–152 (1974).
10. INGRAM, W. T. & GOLDEN, J. Smoke curve calibration. *Journal of the Air Pollution Control Association*, **23**: 110–115 (1973).
11. KRETZSCHMAR, J. G. Comparison between three different methods for the estimation of the total suspended matter in urban air. *Atmospheric environment*, **9**: 931–934 (1975).
12. KRETZSCHMAR, J. G. & PAUWELS, J. B. Comparison between six different instruments to determine suspended particulate matter levels in ambient air. *Science of the total environment*, **23**: 265–272 (1982).
13. PEDACE, E. A. & SANSONE. The relationship between soiling index and suspended particulate matter concentrations. *Journal of the Air Pollution Control Association*, **22**: 348–351 (1972).
14. RENOUX, A. ET AL. Comparison entre deux méthodes de mesure de poids de poussières dans l'air: la gravimétrie et la réflectométrie (SF8) [Comparison

between two methods of measuring the amount of dust in air: gravimetric and reflectometric]. *Pollution Atmosphérique*, **71**: 241–244 (1976).

15. *Air monitoring programme design for urban and industrial areas*. Geneva, World Health Organization, 1977 (Offset Publication No. 33).
16. *Selected methods of measuring air pollutants*. Geneva, World Health Organization, 1976 (Offset Publication No. 24).
17. *Air quality in selected urban areas, 1973–1974*. Geneva, World Health Organization, 1976 (Offset Publication No. 30).
18. *Air quality in selected urban areas, 1975–1976*. Geneva, World Health Organization, 1978 (Offset Publication No. 41).
19. *Sulfur oxides and suspended particulate matter*. Geneva, World Health Organization, 1979 (Environmental Health Criteria No. 8).
20. *Air quality in selected urban areas, 1977–1978*. Geneva, World Health Organization, 1980 (Offset Publication No. 57).
21. *Analysing and interpreting air monitoring data*. Geneva, World Health Organization, 1980 (Offset Publication No. 51).
22. *Air quality in selected urban areas, 1979–1980*. Geneva, World Health Organization, 1983 (Offset Publication No. 76).
23. US Environmental Protection Agency, SAROAD user's manual. Washington, DC, EPA Publication. APTD-0663, 1971.

Annex 1

# Summary of measurement methods[a]

## Methods for determining sulfur dioxide in air

*Flame photometry or gas chromatography–flame photometry*

The flame photometric detector uses a photomultiplier tube to measure the emissions from sulfur compounds introduced into a hydrogen-rich flame. The method can be used either to measure total sulfur (which is generally equivalent to the $SO_2$ concentration in the vicinity of the monitoring station) or $SO_2$ specifically. For specialized applications, in conjunction with gas chromatography, the concentrations of various sulfur-containing compounds in the atmosphere can be determined simultaneously.

*Acidimetric titration method*

In this method, air is bubbled through 0.5 ml/l hydrogen peroxide solution adjusted to pH 4.5. Any sulfur dioxide present forms sulfuric acid, which is titrated against a standard alkali. Usually, an air sample of about 2 $m^3$ per day is bubbled through the solution. Assuming that sulfuric acid is the only acid present, the concentration of sulfur dioxide in the air can be calculated.

*Amperometric or coulometric method*

Air is passed through a cell containing a neutral buffered iodide or bromide electrolyte where an electrical current maintains a constant concentration of free $I_2$ or $Br_2$. When $SO_2$ in the air sample reacts with the $I_2$ or $Br_2$, the change in electrical current necessary to restore or maintain the original concentration of $I_2$ or $Br_2$ is a quantitative measure of the $SO_2$ input. If the rate of the air flowing through the cell is

[a] More complete descriptions of some of these methods are given in: *Selected methods of measuring air pollutants*. Geneva, World Health Organization, 1976 (Offset Publication No. 24).

constant, the $SO_2$ concentration can be related to an electrical signal by dynamic calibration with known $SO_2$ concentration standards.

*Colorimetric method (pararosaniline, TCM, or West-Gaeke method)*

In the instrumental pararosaniline method, $SO_2$ is absorbed continuously in dilute aqueous dipotassium tetrachloromercurate solution to form the non-volatile dichlorosulfitomercurate ion, which then reacts with formaldehyde and bleached pararosaniline to form red-purple pararosaniline methyl sulfonic acid. The sampling rate may vary from 0.2–1.0 litre per minute, depending on the length of the sampling period. This reaction is specific for $SO_2$ and sulfite salts. The colour intensity of the dye, which is proportional to the concentration of $SO_2$, is measured at a wavelength of 560 nm.

*Conductometric method*

Samples are collected at field stations and taken to a central laboratory for conductometric analysis. This analysis is based on the oxidation of $SO_2$ to sulfuric acid by aqueous hydrogen peroxide and the subsequent measurement of the increased electrical conductivity of the solution. Usually, an air sample of about 2 $m^3$ is collected per day. Special precautions should be taken to eliminate other pollutants that could affect the conductivity of the solution (e.g., HCl, $HNO_3$).

*Pulsed fluorescence*

Sulfur dioxide has a fluorescence band centred near 340 nm. This band is sensitive to atmospheric pressure. Current fluorescence $SO_2$ analysers use a pulsed lamp as an excitation source to achieve greater sensitivity. The fluorescence is measured with a photomultiplier and related directly to the concentration of $SO_2$ in the atmosphere.

## Methods for determining suspended particulate matter in air

*High-volume sampler*

Suspended particulate matter is collected by means of a high-volume sampler. The sampler consists of a motor and blower enclosed in a shelter. The filter surface is arranged horizontally, facing upwards, and is protected by a roof that keeps out rain and snow and generally prevents the collection of particles larger than about 100 $\mu m$. Filters are made of glass fibre or synthetic organic fibre. The air flow rates range from 1.1 $m^3$ to 1.7 $m^3$ per minute. The concentration of suspended particulate matter is calculated by dividing the net weight of the particulate matter by the total air volume sampled.

*Tape sampler—transmittance*

The sampler consists of a tape of filter-paper, an intake tube, and a pump. Successive areas of the paper are positioned and clamped between the intake tube and the pump connexion. Air is drawn through the filter for a selected length of time, usually 1–4 hours. An unused portion of the tape is then moved into position and sampling is resumed. The rate of air flow can be regulated and it usually ranges from 4.2 $m^3$ to 5.7 $m^3$ per hour. The samples are evaluated by comparing the transmittance of light through the filter containing the deposit with the transmittance through a clean portion of the filter. In countries where this method is used, transmittance is usually converted into units of coefficient of haze (COH) per thousand linear feet (304.8 m) of air passing through the filter.

*Nephelometry*

Several instruments have been designed for assessing suspended particulate matter by measuring the light scattered by the particles in a given volume of air. The integrating nephelometer draws in a sample of particle-laden air and measures the scattered light over all scattering angles. The measurement is expressed as the "scattering coefficient", which is defined as "the reciprocal of the distance in which 63% of the light is lost from a light beam by scattering". The scattering coefficient is related to visibility ("local visual distance") and, under some conditions, can be related to the mass concentration of suspended particulates when the air is sufficiently dry.

*Smoke-shade method*

When air is drawn through a filter-paper, smoke particles suspended in the air are retained on the paper, forming a stain. "Smoke" is considered to include particles of roughly 10 μm diameter or less. The density of the stain depends partly on the mass of smoke particles collected and partly on the nature of the smoke. The concentration of smoke in the atmosphere can be estimated by drawing a known volume of air through a filter-paper and measuring the density of the resulting stain with a photoelectric reflectometer. Usually, about 2 $m^3$ of air is sampled per day. A calibration curve relating the density of the filter stain to the weight of smoke particles deposited on the filter-paper has been established for "standard urban smoke". Thus, the concentration of smoke per unit volume of air can be calculated and expressed in terms of the "standard smoke" equivalent.

Annex 2

# GEMS quality assurance

## Introduction

Quality assurance is a formalized procedure to help ensure that a monitoring programme will successfully yield data of known quality for the stated monitoring objectives. Since the GEMS network is made up of monitoring sites within participating countries, each with their own quality assurance programme, global efforts have been concentrated on four areas: siting; training; inter-laboratory comparisons; and data validation.

## Siting

The sites of the air quality monitoring stations in each city were chosen by the local staff according to their local/national primary objective for the monitoring data. For example, the sites may have been chosen to represent a large residential area, a suburban industrial complex, or a city-centre commercial district. In order to standardize in a general way the characteristics of each site, a site identification form is required for each station. Provisions are made for specifying the type (industrial, residential, commercial) and the location (city-centre, suburban) of each site. Although not required, a narrative description of each site is often useful, including a description of the major emission sources in the surrounding area and the general topography.

Samplers are usually placed 3–15 metres above ground level, using site exposure criteria common for all stations. Factors that may influence the representativeness of the samples and the interpretation of the resulting data include: variability and intensity of sources; topographical features; meteorological conditions; and demographic features. It is intended that each site should be inspected independently, on a regular basis, to ensure representativeness.

## Training

One of the best ways of ensuring the quality of data is to train staff in such a way that they know how to avoid many of the common errors found in air pollution data. WHO has assisted many developing countries in procuring and installing monitoring equipment and in training staff in its proper operation and maintenance. In addition, WHO has published several publications on the various aspects of air pollution monitoring.[a]

## Inter-laboratory comparisons

Two inter-laboratory comparisons of the measurements of sulfur dioxide concentrations using the pararosaniline (West-Gaeke) method were conducted in 1975 and 1980. In each of these studies, the majority of the results were well within the statistically acceptable range. The major problem, however, was the stability of the test reagent (sodium sulfite) over time and with respect to temperature. Alternative test reagents (reference samples) using the freeze-drying technique are being developed in different laboratories in order to avoid similar problems in future comparisons.

Ambient particles are found in three size classes: the nuclei (Aitken) mode ($< 0.1\ \mu m$); the accumulation mode ($0.1\text{–}2.5\ \mu m$); and the coarse mode ($> 2.5\ \mu m$). The two most common methods for determining ambient particulate concentrations, black smoke by reflectance and total suspended particulates (TSP) determined gravimetrically, collect samples in different size classes: smoke $< 2.5\ \mu m$ and TSP $< 25\ \mu m$. Since there is no standard procedure for generating a reference sample of known concentration, comparisons between measurements made at different locations are useful.

Within the network, comparison studies have been undertaken in Tehran and Copenhagen. The results in Tehran (1980) indicated that the ratio of TSP to smoke was 2 in the lower concentration range and 1.5 in the upper concentration range. At Copenhagen (1978), the corresponding ratio varied between 2 and 2.5. In general, no consistent relationship is to be expected between these two types of observation, since different characteristics of the suspended particulate matter (reflectance and mass) and particles of different sizes are being measured.

These comparison studies are useful in providing a site-specific calibration between smoke and TSP which relates the darkness of the black smoke measurement to the collected mass on the weighed filter. In

---

[a] *Selected methods of measuring air pollutants.* Geneva, World Health Organization, 1976 (Offset Publication No. 24); *Air monitoring programme design for urban and industrial areas.* Geneva, World Health Organization, 1977 (Offset Publication No. 33); *Analysing and interpreting air monitoring data.* Geneva, World Health Organization, 1980 (Offset Publication No. 51).

the absence of a site-specific calibration, the black smoke data if reported in $\mu g/m^3$ are a measure of the mass of a reference smoke that has a standard darkness property. This provides a useful comparison between locations and permits trend analyses over time. It is, however, clear that comparisons of results between locations using different methods for the measurement of suspended particulate matter should be avoided.

## Data validation

Data validation is primarily the responsibility of the reporting country, which has to follow standardized measurement procedures, including quality control checks such as zero and span checks and multipoint calibrations when required. The following discussion pertains to the validation of the data once received by WHO.

The quality of data entering the WHO data collection system is a primary concern. Experience indicates that these data may be subject to various types of error including reporting errors, identification errors, clerical errors, calculation errors, and errors due to anomalous samples, equipment malfunction, etc.

The identification and removal and correction of data with serious errors involves more than the application of automated statistical techniques. The complexity of the types of error which may be present in the data base, the possibility that apparently anomalous values are in fact valid, and the steps required to assess the validity of flagged data all require that the complete validation process be systematized. For example, there are numerous types of spurious data which may be present in a given set of data. There may be either individual observations or entire subsets of the data which are in error. The errors may be completely independent and random, they may be systematic, or they may be correlated in some manner.

The initial procedures for entering and checking data are routine validation procedures which are applied to most data management systems, e.g., duplicate transcription of data followed by cross-checking and format validity tests. These, however, are intended only to identify qualitative errors in the data base. They do not confirm the validity of the reported numerical values for $SO_2$ and SPM.

Acceptance procedures are designed to compare the actual reported data against specified criteria in order to judge the reasonableness of the reported values. These acceptance procedures can identify various types of anomalies (outliers) in the data, including impossible values, individual and multiple outliers and entire subsets of incorrect data.

The basic types of acceptance procedure that are incorporated into the WHO data management system are based on data completeness and gross limit tests. Data completeness tests check whether sufficient data are contained in the data base for statistical analysis and summary purposes. Statistics calculated based on incomplete data are flagged. Other acceptance procedures are also possible, but these are most useful if applied to the data by the originating country. Corrective action, if warranted, will result in more and higher quality data.

**Annex 3**

# WHO Collaborating Centres on air pollution

Australia— WHO Collaborating Centre on Air Pollution Monitoring for the Western Pacific Region, Queensland Air Pollution Control Division, Brisbane
India— WHO Collaborating Centre on Air Pollution for the South-East Asia Region, National Environmental Engineering Institute, Nagpur
Japan— WHO Collaborating Centre on Air Pollution for the Western Pacific Region, Institute of Public Health, Tokyo
Malaysia— Western Pacific Regional Centre for the Promotion of Environmental Planning and Applied Studies, Kuala Lumpur
Peru— Pan American Center for Sanitary Engineering and Environmental Sciences, Lima
Union of Soviet Socialist Republics— WHO Collaborating Centre on Regional Air Pollution Problems, Central Institute for Advanced Medical Training, Moscow
United States of America— WHO Collaborating Centre on Environmental Pollution Control, Environmental Protection Agency, Washington, DC

*National Agencies and Institutes*

Australia— Environmental Protection Agency of Victoria, Melbourne, Victoria
State Pollution Control Commission, Sydney, New South Wales
Belgium— Institute for Hygiene and Epidemiology, Brussels
Brazil— State Foundation for Environmental Engineering (FEEMA), Rio de Janeiro
State Centre for Environmental and Sanitary Technology (CETESB), São Paulo
Canada— Air Pollution Control Directorate, Environment Canada, Ottawa
Chile— Institute for Occupational Health and Air Pollution, Santiago
Colombia— Municipal Health Department, Cali Antioquia Health Service, Medellin District Health Department, Bogota

Cuba—— National Hygiene Directorate, Ministry of Public Health, Havana

Czechoslovakia—— Institute of Hygiene, Prague

Egypt—— Industrial Health Department, Ministry of Health, Cairo

Germany, Federal Republic of—— University Institute of Meteorology and Geophysics, Frankfurt am Main

Hong Kong—— Air Pollution Control Unit, Department of Labour, Hong Kong

Iran (Islamic Republic of)—— Environmental Health Directorate, Ministry of Health and Social Affairs, Tehran

Israel—— Division of Air Pollution and Radiation Control, Ministry of Health, Tel Aviv

Italy—— Division of Air Pollution, Ministry of Health, Rome

The Netherlands—— National Institute of Public Health, Bilthoven

New Zealand—— Air Pollution Control Section, Ministry of Health, Wellington

Peru—— Institute for Occupational Health, Lima

Republic of Korea—— Air Quality Management Bureau, Office of Environment, Seoul

Spain—— Environmental Health Section, National School of Public Health, Madrid

Sweden—— Air Protection Laboratory, National Swedish Environment Protection Board, Nykoping

United Kingdom of Great Britain and Northern Ireland—— Warren Spring Laboratory, Stevenage, Hertfordshire

Venezuela—— Engineering Faculty, Central University of Venezuela, Caracas

Yugoslavia—— Institute of Medical Research and Occupational Health, Zagreb

# Summary of air monitoring project data, 1973–1980

Available number of measurements, yearly averages, 98th percentiles and maximum daily concentrations of $SO_2$ and SPM

(An asterisk indicates that the data set is judged to be not representative for the entire year)

| Country | City | Site No. | Site Area | $SO_2$ Method | | $SO_2$ 73 | 74 | 75 | 76 | 77 | 78 | 79 | 80 | SPM Method | | SPM 73 | 74 | 75 | 76 | 77 | 78 | 79 | 80 |
|---|---|---|---|---|---|---|---|---|---|---|---|---|---|---|---|---|---|---|---|---|---|---|---|
| Australia | Melbourne | 1 | CCC | FPD | *n* | | | 292 | 339 | 312 | 227* | 335 | 295 | Neph | *n* | | | 348 | 352 | 320 | 310 | 284* | |
| | | | | | $\bar{x}$ | | | 16 | 11 | 21 | 12* | 4 | 7 | | $\bar{x}$ | | | 28 | 26 | 24 | 30 | 21* | |
| | | | | | $P_{98}$ | | | 47 | 37 | 52 | 26* | 26 | 26 | | $P_{98}$ | | | 120 | 63 | 60 | 108 | 72* | |
| | | | | | max | | | 105 | 50 | 79 | 52* | 50 | 26 | | max | | | 225 | 180 | 81 | 189 | 123* | |
| | | | | | | | | | | | | | | Hi-vol | *n* | | | | | | 54 | 46 | |
| | | | | | | | | | | | | | | | $\bar{x}$ | | | | | | 71 | 73 | |
| | | | | | | | | | | | | | | | $P_{98}$ | | | | | | 134 | 126 | |
| | | | | | | | | | | | | | | | max | | | | | | 142 | 129 | |
| | Sydney | 1 | CCC | Acid | *n* | | | 242* | 341 | 271* | 325 | 330 | 361 | Hi-vol | *n* | | | 42* | 61 | 58 | 55 | 58 | 55 |
| | | | | | $\bar{x}$ | | | 73* | 70 | 74* | 63 | 46 | 61 | | $\bar{x}$ | | | 98* | 92 | 92 | 95 | 100 | 118 |
| | | | | | $P_{98}$ | | | 135* | 113 | 136* | 154 | 95 | 160 | | $P_{98}$ | | | 184* | 145 | 151 | 214 | 183 | 186 |
| | | | | | max | | | 159* | 152 | 151* | 246 | 115 | 255 | | max | | | 200* | 202 | 163 | 246 | 316 | 462 |
| | | 2 | SR | Acid | *n* | | | 364 | 363 | 255* | 291 | 324 | 114* | Hi-vol | *n* | | | 53 | 60 | 57 | 56 | 54 | 24* |
| | | | | | $\bar{x}$ | | | 44 | 42 | 41* | 37 | 22 | 28* | | $\bar{x}$ | | | 76 | 74 | 81 | 72 | 81 | 75* |
| | | | | | $P_{98}$ | | | 78 | 71 | 75* | 113 | 50 | 75* | | $P_{98}$ | | | 163 | 128 | 177 | 118 | 162 | 116* |
| | | | | | max | | | 89 | 77 | 83* | 150 | 100 | 105* | | max | | | 360 | 142 | 183 | 125 | 192 | 116* |
| | | 3 | SI | Acid | *n* | | | 340 | 354 | 241* | 336 | 322 | 343 | Hi-vol | *n* | | | 50 | 58 | 51 | 53 | 56 | 56 |
| | | | | | $\bar{x}$ | | | 31 | 30 | 27* | 19 | 29 | 43 | | $\bar{x}$ | | | 156 | 89 | 102 | 108 | 85 | 85 |
| | | | | | $P_{98}$ | | | 58 | 44 | 53* | 60 | 70 | 110 | | $P_{98}$ | | | 567 | 162 | 203 | 215 | 147 | 171 |
| | | | | | max | | | 112 | 58 | 80* | 90 | 165 | 225 | | max | | | 657 | 226 | 224 | 339 | 162 | 182 |

Annex 4 (*cont.*)

| Country | City | Site No. | Site Area | SO2 Method | | SO2 73 | 74 | 75 | 76 | 77 | 78 | 79 | 80 | SPM Method | | SPM 73 | 74 | 75 | 76 | 77 | 78 | 79 | 80 |
|---|---|---|---|---|---|---|---|---|---|---|---|---|---|---|---|---|---|---|---|---|---|---|---|
| Belgium | Brussels | 1 | CCC | Acid | $n$ | 277 | 355 | 326 | 240* | 344 | 337 | 363 | 356 | Smoke | $n$ | 282 | 357 | 328 | 247* | 344 | 344 | 363 | 364 |
| | | | | | $\bar{x}$ | 121 | 107 | 87 | 115* | 88 | 101 | 96 | 76 | | $\bar{x}$ | 38 | 28 | 32 | 31* | 24 | 29 | 27 | 19 |
| | | | | | $P_{98}$ | 342 | 232 | 351 | 324* | 309 | 267 | 349 | 200 | | $P_{98}$ | 109 | 72 | 114 | 85* | 64 | 96 | 92 | 51 |
| | | | | | max | 608 | 346 | 526 | 374* | 740 | 349 | 614 | 327 | | max | 175 | 106 | 417 | 163* | 203 | 126 | 159 | 92 |
| | | 2 | SR | Acid | $n$ | 323 | 213* | 348 | 344 | 317 | 355 | 331 | 328 | Smoke | $n$ | 323 | 213* | 348 | 351 | 318 | 355 | 338 | 344 |
| | | | | | $\bar{x}$ | 101 | 85* | 87 | 87 | 67 | 70 | 75 | 69 | | $\bar{x}$ | 30 | 19* | 26 | 23 | 17 | 17 | 20 | 17 |
| | | | | | $P_{98}$ | 285 | 204* | 270 | 248 | 174 | 187 | 215 | 199 | | $P_{98}$ | 71 | 59* | 89 | 72 | 43 | 47 | 57 | 53 |
| | | | | | max | 411 | 251* | 460 | 323 | 251 | 277 | 347 | 359 | | max | 107 | 75* | 205 | 87 | 112 | 72 | 72 | 90 |
| | | 3 | SI | Acid | $n$ | 276 | 319 | 363 | 295 | 317 | 346 | 301 | 365 | Smoke | $n$ | 283 | 319 | 364 | 309 | 317 | 347 | 301 | 365 |
| | | | | | $\bar{x}$ | 119 | 107 | 99 | 94 | 79 | 60 | 84 | 64 | | $\bar{x}$ | 26 | 23 | 27 | 21 | 14 | 11 | 17 | 15 |
| | | | | | $P_{98}$ | 274 | 257 | 260 | 222 | 177 | 117 | 205 | 186 | | $P_{98}$ | 83 | 63 | 96 | 64 | 54 | 42 | 60 | 47 |
| | | | | | max | 469 | 439 | 518 | 316 | 331 | 213 | 404 | 272 | | max | 124 | 95 | 190 | 99 | 78 | 105 | 132 | 77 |
| Brazil | Rio de Janeiro | 1 | CCC | Acid | $n$ | | | | 214 | 215 | 67* | | | Smoke | $n$ | | | | 214 | 99* | 67* | | |
| | | | | | $\bar{x}$ | | | | 57 | 128 | 208* | | | | $\bar{x}$ | | | | 31 | 33* | 19* | | |
| | | | | | $P_{98}$ | | | | 132 | 677 | 927* | | | | $P_{98}$ | | | | 75 | 98* | 75* | | |
| | | | | | max | | | | 203 | 891 | 965* | | | | max | | | | 113 | 98* | 92* | | |
| | São Paulo | 2 | CCC | Acid | $n$ | | | | 365 | 364 | 303 | 364 | 365 | Smoke | $n$ | | | | 366 | 364 | 303 | 365 | 365 |
| | | | | | $\bar{x}$ | | | | 106 | 126 | 125 | 153 | 135 | | $\bar{x}$ | | | | 98 | 89 | 81 | 85 | 80 |
| | | | | | $P_{98}$ | | | | 291 | 300 | 283 | 403 | 332 | | $P_{98}$ | | | | 340 | 248 | 252 | 268 | 221 |
| | | | | | max | | | | 340 | 388 | 351 | 466 | 483 | | max | | | | 447 | 304 | 301 | 333 | 291 |
| | | 3 | CCI | Acid | $n$ | | | | 365 | 364 | 302 | 360 | 358 | Smoke | $n$ | | | | 364 | 364 | 302 | 360 | 359 |
| | | | | | $\bar{x}$ | | | | 122 | 115 | 111 | 135 | 113 | | $\bar{x}$ | | | | 88 | 72 | 68 | 70 | 61 |
| | | | | | $P_{98}$ | | | | 284 | 214 | 211 | 304 | 236 | | $P_{98}$ | | | | 342 | 242 | 248 | 228 | 199 |
| | | | | | max | | | | 341 | 256 | 258 | 405 | 374 | | max | | | | 666 | 287 | 288 | 419 | 369 |
| | | 4 | CCR | Acid | $n$ | | | | 362 | 364 | 299 | 365 | 356 | Smoke | $n$ | | | | 362 | 364 | 299 | 364 | 356 |
| | | | | | $\bar{x}$ | | | | 72 | 84 | 93 | 111 | 105 | | $\bar{x}$ | | | | 84 | 79 | 74 | 72 | 70 |
| | | | | | $P_{98}$ | | | | 156 | 168 | 201 | 234 | 223 | | $P_{98}$ | | | | 273 | 198 | 213 | 208 | 195 |
| | | | | | max | | | | 212 | 233 | 227 | 316 | 294 | | max | | | | 381 | 267 | 266 | 244 | 241 |

| | | | | | | | | | | | | | | | | | | | | | | |
|---|---|---|---|---|---|---|---|---|---|---|---|---|---|---|---|---|---|---|---|---|---|---|
| Canada | Hamilton | 1 | SR | Coul | $n$ | | | | 346 | 350 | 348 | 357 | 345 | Hi-vol | $n$ | | | | 53 | 54 | 55 | 51 | 55 |
| | | | | | $\bar{x}$ | | | | 52 | 43 | 34 | 32 | 35 | | $\bar{x}$ | | | | 114 | 108 | 99 | 114 | 112 |
| | | | | | $P_{98}$ | | | | 157 | 131 | 131 | 131 | 131 | | $P_{98}$ | | | | 267 | 216 | 196 | 232 | 228 |
| | | | | | max | | | | 288 | 210 | 183 | 210 | 183 | | max | | | | 273 | 222 | 212 | 241 | 255 |
| | | 2 | CCC | Coul | $n$ | | | | 363 | 363 | 362 | 363 | 365 | Hi-vol | $n$ | | | | 48 | 52 | 49 | 56 | 56 |
| | | | | | $\bar{x}$ | | | | 53 | 57 | 39 | 42 | 32 | | $\bar{x}$ | | | | 121 | 103 | 124 | 121 | 99 |
| | | | | | $P_{98}$ | | | | 183 | 183 | 157 | 157 | 131 | | $P_{98}$ | | | | 335 | 243 | 267 | 360 | 190 |
| | | | | | max | | | | 236 | 210 | 183 | 262 | 157 | | max | | | | 541 | 483 | 270 | 801 | 227 |
| | Montreal | 1 | SR | Coul | $n$ | | | | 358 | 362 | 351 | 287 | 290 | Hi-vol | $n$ | | | | 50 | 56 | 55 | 53 | 49 |
| | | | | | $\bar{x}$ | | | | 14 | 41 | 27 | 30 | 24 | | $\bar{x}$ | | | | 92 | 73 | 70 | 68 | 75 |
| | | | | | $P_{98}$ | | | | LD | 183 | 131 | 131 | 105 | | $P_{98}$ | | | | 168 | 149 | 171 | 138 | 166 |
| | | | | | max | | | | 52 | 314 | 262 | 210 | 183 | | max | | | | 184 | 164 | 194 | 138 | 171 |
| | | 2 | SR | Coul | $n$ | | | | 342 | 331 | 272 | 293 | 242* | Hi-vol | $n$ | | | | 52 | 58 | 56 | 59 | 60 |
| | | | | | $\bar{x}$ | | | | 59 | 55 | 71 | 47 | 37* | | $\bar{x}$ | | | | 76 | 77 | 74 | 73 | 84 |
| | | | | | $P_{98}$ | | | | 210 | 236 | 236 | 210 | 157* | | $P_{98}$ | | | | 137 | 166 | 170 | 186 | 199 |
| | | | | | max | | | | 288 | 367 | 288 | 262 | 183* | | max | | | | 138 | 184 | 192 | 195 | 218 |
| | | 3 | CCC | Coul | $n$ | | | | 321 | 325 | 320 | 318 | 302 | Hi-vol | $n$ | | | | | 56 | 58 | 62 | 56 |
| | | | | | $\bar{x}$ | | | | 59 | 45 | 45 | 44 | 40 | | $\bar{x}$ | | | | | 68 | 64 | 64 | 69 |
| | | | | | $P_{98}$ | | | | 210 | 210 | 157 | 157 | 131 | | $P_{98}$ | | | | | 139 | 134 | 143 | 127 |
| | | | | | max | | | | 288 | 341 | 183 | 210 | 210 | | max | | | | | 184 | 207 | 159 | 146 |
| | Toronto | 1 | SI | Coul | $n$ | | | | 322 | 330 | 345 | 344 | 333 | Hi-vol | $n$ | | | | 48 | 57 | 58 | 61 | 58 |
| | | | | | $\bar{x}$ | | | | 23 | 26 | 22 | 18 | 19 | | $\bar{x}$ | | | | 82 | 70 | 76 | 90 | 99 |
| | | | | | $P_{98}$ | | | | 105 | 105 | 79 | 79 | 52 | | $P_{98}$ | | | | 185 | 130 | 140 | 166 | 199 |
| | | | | | max | | | | 183 | 183 | 131 | 131 | 131 | | max | | | | 260 | 140 | 147 | 196 | 209 |
| | | 2 | SR | Coul | $n$ | | | | 347 | 348 | 345 | 329 | 341 | Hi-vol | $n$ | | | | 52 | 61 | 54 | 58 | 57 |
| | | | | | $\bar{x}$ | | | | 34 | 32 | 20 | 24 | 22 | | $\bar{x}$ | | | | 71 | 66 | 66 | 76 | 76 |
| | | | | | $P_{98}$ | | | | 131 | 131 | 105 | 79 | 79 | | $P_{98}$ | | | | 145 | 127 | 129 | 166 | 135 |
| | | | | | max | | | | 157 | 183 | 183 | 105 | 236 | | max | | | | 154 | 203 | 167 | 171 | 153 |
| | | 3 | CCC | Coul | $n$ | | | | 362 | 362 | 362 | 361 | 363 | Hi-vol | $n$ | | | | 55 | 57 | 51 | 52 | 57 |
| | | | | | $\bar{x}$ | | | | 35 | 35 | 27 | 23 | 20 | | $\bar{x}$ | | | | 70 | 75 | 73 | 84 | 79 |
| | | | | | $P_{98}$ | | | | 105 | 131 | 105 | 79 | 79 | | $P_{98}$ | | | | 159 | 162 | 167 | 175 | 178 |
| | | | | | max | | | | 157 | 210 | 236 | 210 | 131 | | max | | | | 173 | 179 | 168 | 185 | 178 |

Annex 4 (*cont.*)

| Country | City | Site | | | SO2 | | | | | | | | | SPM | | | | | | | | | |
|---|---|---|---|---|---|---|---|---|---|---|---|---|---|---|---|---|---|---|---|---|---|---|---|
| | | | | | | Year | | | | | | | | | | Year | | | | | | | |
| | | No. | Area | Method | | 73 | 74 | 75 | 76 | 77 | 78 | 79 | 80 | Method | | 73 | 74 | 75 | 76 | 77 | 78 | 79 | 80 |
| Canada (*cont.*) | Vancouver | 1 | CCC | Coul | $n$ | 344 | 274 | | | | | | | Hi-vol | $n$ | 51 | 56 | 28* | | | | | |
| | | | | | $\bar{x}$ | 21 | 20 | | | | | | | | $\bar{x}$ | 65 | 64 | 57* | | | | | |
| | | | | | $P_{98}$ | 74 | 55 | | | | | | | | $P_{98}$ | 124 | 129 | 84* | | | | | |
| | | | | | max | 205 | 87 | | | | | | | | max | 131 | 134 | 161* | | | | | |
| | | 2 | CCR | Coul | $n$ | 353 | 278 | 270 | 214* | 116* | 247* | 255* | 307 | Hi-vol | $n$ | 58 | 54 | 60 | 37* | 57 | 59 | 53 | 51 |
| | | | | | $\bar{x}$ | 21 | 18 | 20 | 18* | 19* | 17* | 18* | 16 | | $\bar{x}$ | 64 | 64 | 66 | 64* | 62 | 52 | 70 | 62 |
| | | | | | $P_{98}$ | 73 | 60 | 70 | 61* | 79* | 79* | 79* | 52 | | $P_{98}$ | 133 | 124 | 179 | 142* | 168 | 135 | 203 | 105 |
| | | | | | max | 227 | 85 | 166 | 75* | 79* | 79* | 79* | 79 | | max | 136 | 127 | 234 | 146* | 170 | 179 | 213 | 178 |
| | | 4 | SI | Coul | $n$ | 141* | 339 | 228* | 231* | 89* | 163* | 267* | 96* | Hi-vol | $n$ | 21* | 59 | 50 | 49 | 54 | 59 | 60 | 52 |
| | | | | | $\bar{x}$ | 14* | 14 | 14* | 14* | 13* | 14* | 17* | 13* | | $\bar{x}$ | 78* | 75 | 60 | 77 | 90 | 90 | 97 | 79 |
| | | | | | $P_{98}$ | 37* | LD | 37* | 33* | LD* | 52* | 52* | LD* | | $P_{98}$ | 155* | 181 | 154 | 179 | 209 | 168 | 256 | 150 |
| | | | | | max | 51* | 62 | 60* | 52* | 13* | 52* | 52* | 13* | | max | 155* | 271 | 175 | 182 | 223 | 223 | 276 | 272 |
| | | 5 | CCC | Coul | $n$ | | | 264 | 329 | 248* | 100* | 273 | | Hi-vol | $n$ | | | 17* | 59 | 58 | 59 | 58 | 51 |
| | | | | | $\bar{x}$ | | | 29 | 25 | 21* | 19* | 18 | | | $\bar{x}$ | | | 67* | 74 | 76 | 72 | 69 | 76 |
| | | | | | $P_{98}$ | | | 98 | 79 | 79* | 52* | 19 | | | $P_{98}$ | | | 148* | 130 | 191 | 150 | 168 | 144 |
| | | | | | max | | | 160 | 114 | 157* | 79* | 105 | | | max | | | 148* | 183 | 202 | 203 | 188 | 166 |
| Chile | Santiago | 1 | CCC | Acid | $n$ | | | | 347 | 318 | 358 | 216* | 319 | Smoke | $n$ | | | | 276* | 345 | 356 | 211* | 313 |
| | | | | | $\bar{x}$ | | | | 72 | 62 | 93 | 54* | 58 | | $\bar{x}$ | | | | 72* | 85 | 115 | 68* | 100 |
| | | | | | $P_{98}$ | | | | 198 | 179 | 254 | 203* | 169 | | $P_{98}$ | | | | 240* | 315 | 316 | 237* | 363 |
| | | | | | max | | | | 277 | 232 | 360 | 213* | 441 | | max | | | | 612* | 354 | 475 | 529* | 404 |
| | | 2 | CCR | Acid | $n$ | | | | 324 | 295* | 329 | 262* | 244* | Smoke | $n$ | | | | 329 | 318 | 313 | 202* | 246* |
| | | | | | $\bar{x}$ | | | | 48 | 43* | 51 | 56* | 40* | | $\bar{x}$ | | | | 68 | 25 | 36 | 63* | 40* |
| | | | | | $P_{98}$ | | | | 128 | 133* | 168 | 178* | 133* | | $P_{98}$ | | | | 374 | 153 | 196 | 359* | 143* |
| | | | | | max | | | | 192 | 480* | 179 | 239* | 266* | | max | | | | 497 | 306 | 272 | 526* | 353* |
| | | 3 | CCC | Acid | $n$ | | | | | 97 | | 38* | | Smoke | $n$ | | | | | 97 | | 38* | |
| | | | | | $\bar{x}$ | | | | | 59 | | 137* | | | $\bar{x}$ | | | | | 63 | | 65* | |
| | | | | | $P_{98}$ | | | | | 161 | | 256* | | | $P_{98}$ | | | | | 194 | | 144* | |
| | | | | | max | | | | | 304 | | 320* | | | max | | | | | 216 | | 146* | |

| | | | | | | | | | | | | | |
|---|---|---|---|---|---|---|---|---|---|---|---|---|---|
| Colombia | Bogota | 1 | CCC | Acid | $n$ | | | | 307 | 313 | 119* | 44* | 22* |
| | | | | | $\bar{x}$ | | | | 18 | 15 | 13* | 4* | 3* |
| | | | | | $P_{98}$ | | | | 41 | 36 | 31* | 12* | 7* |
| | | | | | max | | | | 271 | 45 | 35* | 23* | 7* |
| | | 2 | SR | Acid | $n$ | | | | 151* | 94* | | | |
| | | | | | $\bar{x}$ | | | | 25* | 20* | | | |
| | | | | | $P_{98}$ | | | | 59* | 48* | | | |
| | | | | | max | | | | 66* | 49* | | | |
| | | 3 | SI | Acid | $n$ | | | | 226* | 46* | 56* | 93* | 32* |
| | | | | | $\bar{x}$ | | | | 95* | 24* | 87* | 68* | 11* |
| | | | | | $P_{98}$ | | | | 150* | 34* | 174* | 152* | 40* |
| | | | | | max | | | | 191* | 40* | 235* | 168* | 48* |
| | Cali | 1 | SI | Acid | $n$ | | | | 165 | 14* | | 22* | 21* |
| | | | | | $\bar{x}$ | | | | 21 | 7* | | 40* | 9* |
| | | | | | $P_{98}$ | | | | 56 | 18* | | 170* | 88* |
| | | | | | max | | | | 64 | 18* | | 170* | 88* |
| | | 2 | CCC | Acid | $n$ | | | | 131* | 35* | | | |
| | | | | | $\bar{x}$ | | | | 8* | 14* | | | |
| | | | | | $P_{98}$ | | | | 24* | 27* | | | |
| | | | | | max | | | | 29* | 66* | | | |
| | Medellin | 3 | SR | Acid | $n$ | | | | 179 | 114 | | 37* | 33* |
| | | | | | $\bar{x}$ | | | | 6 | 10 | | 14* | 4* |
| | | | | | $P_{98}$ | | | | 23 | 36 | | 43* | 16* |
| | | | | | max | | | | 41 | 65 | | 55* | 32* |
| | | 1 | SR | Acid | $n$ | | | | 260 | | 102 | 129 | |
| | | | | | $\bar{x}$ | | | | 25 | | 16 | 34 | |
| | | | | | $P_{98}$ | | | | 55 | | 34 | 80 | |
| | | | | | max | | | | 219 | | 36 | 93 | |

| | | | | | | | | | | | | | |
|---|---|---|---|---|---|---|---|---|---|---|---|---|---|
| Colombia | Bogota | 1 | CCC | Smoke | $n$ | | | | 270 | 323 | 122* | 44* | 31* |
| | | | | | $\bar{x}$ | | | | 32 | 24 | 19* | 9* | 10* |
| | | | | | $P_{98}$ | | | | 70 | 82 | 55* | 35* | 30* |
| | | | | | max | | | | 339 | 101 | 111* | 36* | 33* |
| | | 2 | SR | Smoke | $n$ | | | | 183* | 101* | | | |
| | | | | | $\bar{x}$ | | | | 56* | 42* | | | |
| | | | | | $P_{98}$ | | | | 177* | 73* | | | |
| | | | | | max | | | | 215* | 108* | | | |
| | | 3 | SI | Smoke | $n$ | | | | 202* | 53* | 56* | 95* | 32* |
| | | | | | $\bar{x}$ | | | | 94* | 50* | 171* | 172* | 120* |
| | | | | | $P_{98}$ | | | | 236* | 96* | 415* | 620* | 198* |
| | | | | | max | | | | 306* | 111* | 496* | 677* | 202* |
| | Cali | 1 | SI | Smoke | $n$ | | | | 165 | 25* | | 22* | 21* |
| | | | | | $\bar{x}$ | | | | 55 | 45* | | 28* | 21* |
| | | | | | $P_{98}$ | | | | 110 | 92* | | 44* | 62* |
| | | | | | max | | | | 129 | 92* | | 44* | 62* |
| | | 2 | CCC | Smoke | $n$ | | | | 133* | 35* | | | |
| | | | | | $\bar{x}$ | | | | 26* | 26* | | | |
| | | | | | $P_{98}$ | | | | 44* | 89* | | | |
| | | | | | max | | | | 73* | 93* | | | |
| | Medellin | 3 | SR | Smoke | $n$ | | | | 183 | 125 | | 37* | 39* |
| | | | | | $\bar{x}$ | | | | 22 | 27 | | 20* | 10* |
| | | | | | $P_{98}$ | | | | 43 | 99 | | 77* | 12* |
| | | | | | max | | | | 84 | 288 | | 109* | 42* |
| | | 1 | SR | Smoke | $n$ | | | | 265 | | 102 | 129 | |
| | | | | | $\bar{x}$ | | | | 44 | | 21 | 56 | |
| | | | | | $P_{98}$ | | | | 116 | | 43 | 112 | |
| | | | | | max | | | | 381 | | 50 | 1041 | |

Annex 4 (*cont.*)

| Country | City | Site | | SO₂ | | | | | | | | | | SPM | | | | | | | | | |
|---|---|---|---|---|---|---|---|---|---|---|---|---|---|---|---|---|---|---|---|---|---|---|---|
| | | | | | | Year | | | | | | | | | | Year | | | | | | | |
| | | No. | Area | Method | | 73 | 74 | 75 | 76 | 77 | 78 | 79 | 80 | Method | | 73 | 74 | 75 | 76 | 77 | 78 | 79 | 80 |
| Cuba | Havana | 1 | CCC | Acid | $n$ | | | | 331 | 336 | 291 | 208* | | Smoke | $n$ | | | | 317 | 337 | 291 | 207* | |
| | | | | | $\bar{x}$ | | | | 66 | 58 | 51 | 48* | | | $\bar{x}$ | | | | 46 | 49 | 56 | 43* | |
| | | | | | $P_{98}$ | | | | 127 | 131 | 104 | 123* | | | $P_{98}$ | | | | 118 | 111 | 117 | 121* | |
| | | | | | max | | | | 180 | 263 | 138 | 249* | | | max | | | | 307 | 218 | 142 | 161* | |
| | | 2 | CCI | Acid | $n$ | | | | 332 | 323 | 305 | 225* | | Smoke | $n$ | | | | 346 | 323 | 309 | 225* | |
| | | | | | $\bar{x}$ | | | | 31 | 22 | 22 | 22* | | | $\bar{x}$ | | | | 61 | 59 | 50 | 101* | |
| | | | | | $P_{98}$ | | | | 71 | 91 | 97 | 70* | | | $P_{98}$ | | | | 200 | 139 | 166 | 346* | |
| | | | | | max | | | | 138 | 537 | 221 | 408* | | | max | | | | 323 | 228 | 399 | 761* | |
| | | 3 | CCR | Acid | $n$ | | | | 312 | 343 | 327 | 221* | | Smoke | $n$ | | | | 320 | 343 | 328 | 221* | |
| | | | | | $x$ | | | | 42 | 29 | 44 | 35* | | | $\bar{x}$ | | | | 28 | 25 | 41 | 49* | |
| | | | | | $P_{98}$ | | | | 133 | 110 | 117 | 94* | | | $P_{98}$ | | | | 81 | 80 | 109 | 178* | |
| | | | | | max | | | | 199 | 180 | 285 | 122* | | | max | | | | 110 | 138 | 218 | 378* | |
| Czecho-slovakia | Prague | 1 | CCC | TCM | $n$ | 358 | 363 | 363 | 360 | 326 | 166* | | | Membrane grav sampler | $n$ | | 126* | 237 | 238 | 202 | 107* | | |
| | | | | | $\bar{x}$ | 148 | 126 | 138 | 130 | 140 | 154* | | | | $\bar{x}$ | | 239* | 262 | 143 | 158 | 136* | | |
| | | | | | $P_{98}$ | 480 | 348 | 486 | 414 | 411 | 381* | | | | $P_{98}$ | | 530* | 880 | 320 | 550 | 355* | | |
| | | | | | max | 874 | 462 | 704 | 602 | 607 | 516* | | | | max | | 735* | 1200 | 375 | 755 | 382* | | |
| | | 2 | SR | TCM | $n$ | 335 | 336 | 360 | 350 | 345 | 181* | | | Membrane grav sampler | $n$ | 335 | 319 | 348 | 354 | 344 | 181* | | |
| | | | | | $\bar{x}$ | 126 | 107 | 129 | 110 | 131 | 129* | | | | $\bar{x}$ | 139 | 135 | 138 | 124 | 125 | 115* | | |
| | | | | | $P_{98}$ | 381 | 272 | 421 | 316 | 447 | 376* | | | | $P_{98}$ | 366 | 414 | 345 | 291 | 315 | 256* | | |
| | | | | | max | 683 | 531 | 619 | 411 | 857 | 480* | | | | max | 758 | 529 | 599 | 399 | 570 | 311* | | |
| | | 3 | CCI | TCM | $n$ | 250 | 226 | 276 | 231 | 280 | 172* | | | Membrane grav sampler | $n$ | | 116* | 235 | 176* | 223 | 105* | | |
| | | | | | $\bar{x}$ | 75 | 56 | 58 | 71 | 67 | 64* | | | | $\bar{x}$ | | 121* | 191 | 132* | 154 | 118* | | |
| | | | | | $P_{98}$ | 260 | 177 | 246 | 223 | 236 | 180* | | | | $P_{98}$ | | 250* | 555 | 295* | 561 | 342* | | |
| | | | | | max | 377 | 267 | 412 | 273 | 459 | 237* | | | | max | | 355* | 929 | 370* | 835 | 634* | | |

| | | | | | | | | | | | | | | | | | | | | | | | |
|---|---|---|---|---|---|---|---|---|---|---|---|---|---|---|---|---|---|---|---|---|---|---|---|
| Denmark | Copen-hagen | 1 | CCC | Acid | $n$<br>$\bar{x}$<br>$P_{98}$<br>max | | | | | 168<br>53<br>131<br>192 | 228<br>30<br>150<br>202 | 176<br>27<br>102<br>300 | 191<br>21<br>84<br>318 | Hi-vol | $n$<br>$\bar{x}$<br>$P_{98}$<br>max | | | | | 348<br>30<br>85<br>149 | 365<br>35<br>87<br>129 | 355<br>33<br>81<br>125 | 349<br>31<br>77<br>111 |
| | | | | | | | | | | | | | | Smoke | $n$<br>$\bar{x}$<br>$P_{98}$<br>max | | | | | 365<br>15<br>34<br>48 | 350<br>14<br>35<br>45 | 354<br>16<br>47<br>63 | 364<br>24<br>57<br>66 |
| | | 2 | SC | Acid | $n$<br>$\bar{x}$<br>$P_{98}$<br>max | | | | | 174<br>37<br>150<br>595 | 195<br>18<br>70<br>212 | 174<br>13<br>61<br>135 | 192<br>16<br>78<br>109 | Hi-vol | $n$<br>$\bar{x}$<br>$P_{98}$<br>max | | | | | 359<br>27<br>64<br>97 | 327<br>36<br>73<br>124 | 339<br>32<br>78<br>120 | 348<br>30<br>72<br>101 |
| | | | | | | | | | | | | | | Smoke | $n$<br>$\bar{x}$<br>$P_{98}$<br>max | | | | | 336<br>8<br>20<br>30 | 330<br>9<br>24<br>35 | 340<br>10<br>17<br>70 | 364<br>14<br>23<br>57 |
| | | 3 | SI | Acid | $n$<br>$\bar{x}$<br>$P_{98}$<br>max | | | | | | 66*<br>23*<br>90*<br>117* | 177<br>32<br>172<br>413 | 186<br>26<br>105<br>141 | Hi-vol | $n$<br>$\bar{x}$<br>$P_{98}$<br>max | | | | | | 132*<br>43*<br>90*<br>108* | 348<br>52<br>143<br>183 | 346<br>45<br>116<br>222 |
| | | | | | | | | | | | | | | Smoke | $n$<br>$\bar{x}$<br>$P_{98}$<br>max | | | | | 361<br>10<br>26<br>41 | 364<br>10<br>29<br>41 | 340<br>11<br>36<br>53 | 364<br>16<br>49<br>78 |
| Egypt | Cairo | 1 | CCC | Acid | $n$<br>$\bar{x}$<br>$P_{98}$<br>max | | | 340<br>61<br>155<br>212 | 301<br>69<br>181<br>259 | 287*<br>39*<br>110*<br>157* | | | 51*<br>7*<br>70*<br>78* | Smoke | $n$<br>$\bar{x}$<br>$P_{98}$<br>max | | | 339<br>64<br>229<br>330 | 296<br>70<br>190<br>364 | 287<br>47<br>165<br>181 | | | 44*<br>101*<br>261*<br>291* |
| | | 2 | SI | Acid | $n$<br>$\bar{x}$<br>$P_{98}$<br>max | | | | 87*<br>40*<br>122*<br>131* | 185*<br>16*<br>58*<br>65* | 55*<br>68*<br>251*<br>280* | | | Smoke | $n$<br>$\bar{x}$<br>$P_{98}$<br>max | | | | 72*<br>105*<br>239*<br>300* | 239<br>64<br>201<br>239 | 55*<br>105*<br>245*<br>269* | | |
| | | 3 | SR | Acid | $n$<br>$\bar{x}$<br>$P_{98}$<br>max | | | | 73*<br>40*<br>121*<br>121* | 135*<br>27*<br>138*<br>163* | 20*<br>14*<br>60*<br>113* | | 14*<br>2*<br>LD*<br>3* | Smoke | $n$<br>$x$<br>$P_{98}$<br>max | | | | 82*<br>55*<br>148*<br>304* | 125*<br>49*<br>196*<br>260* | 22*<br>72*<br>169*<br>169* | | 17*<br>83*<br>172*<br>172* |

Annex 4 (*cont.*)

| Country | City | Site | | SO$_2$ | | | | | | | | | | SPM | | | | | | | | | |
|---|---|---|---|---|---|---|---|---|---|---|---|---|---|---|---|---|---|---|---|---|---|---|---|
| | | No. | Area | Method | | Year 73 | 74 | 75 | 76 | 77 | 78 | 79 | 80 | Method | | Year 73 | 74 | 75 | 76 | 77 | 78 | 79 | 80 |
| Finland | Helsinki | 1 | CCC | Coul | *n* | | | | | | 353 | 356 | 347 | Hi-vol | *n* | | | | | | 148 | 171 | 167 |
| | | | | | $\bar{x}$ | | | | | | 25 | 24 | 27 | | $\bar{x}$ | | | | | | 67 | 64 | 75 |
| | | | | | $P_{98}$ | | | | | | 101 | 77 | 101 | | $P_{98}$ | | | | | | 150 | 162 | 348 |
| | | | | | max | | | | | | 158 | 128 | 128 | | max | | | | | | 267 | 235 | 395 |
| | | 2 | SI | Coul | *n* | | | | | | 354 | 338 | 345 | Hi-vol | *n* | | | | | | 174 | 165 | 161 |
| | | | | | $\bar{x}$ | | | | | | 29 | 28 | 33 | | $\bar{x}$ | | | | | | 57 | 62 | 76 |
| | | | | | $P_{98}$ | | | | | | 104 | 128 | 134 | | $P_{98}$ | | | | | | 132 | 170 | 219 |
| | | | | | max | | | | | | 136 | 211 | 182 | | max | | | | | | 237 | 271 | 312 |
| | | 3 | CCR | Coul | *n* | | | | | | 348 | 253 | 357 | | *n* | | | | | | 174 | 167 | 171 |
| | | | | | $\bar{x}$ | | | | | | 26 | 26 | 30 | | $\bar{x}$ | | | | | | 144 | 124 | 163 |
| | | | | | $P_{98}$ | | | | | | 123 | 104 | 142 | | $P_{98}$ | | | | | | 599 | 733 | 906 |
| | | | | | max | | | | | | 318 | 211 | 192 | | max | | | | | | 1113 | 1051 | 1451 |
| France | Gourdon (Paris) | 1 | SI | Acid | *n* | | | | | 364 | 364 | 364 | 364 | Smoke | *n* | | | | | 364 | 365 | 365 | 366 |
| | | | | | $\bar{x}$ | | | | | 122 | 131 | 105 | 95 | | $\bar{x}$ | | | | | 38 | 41 | 41 | 40 |
| | | | | | $P_{98}$ | | | | | 404 | 352 | 403 | 270 | | $P_{98}$ | | | | | 110 | 148 | 141 | 116 |
| | | | | | max | | | | | 851 | 485 | 547 | 466 | | max | | | | | 432 | 211 | 222 | 220 |
| | | 2 | CCC | Acid | *n* | | | | | 365 | | | | Smoke | *n* | | | | | 365 | | | |
| | | | | | $\bar{x}$ | | | | | 77 | | | | | $\bar{x}$ | | | | | 47 | | | |
| | | | | | $P_{98}$ | | | | | 290 | | | | | $P_{98}$ | | | | | 140 | | | |
| | | | | | max | | | | | 431 | | | | | max | | | | | 274 | | | |
| | | 3 | CCR | Acid | *n* | | | | | 361 | | 354 | 360 | Smoke | *n* | | | | | 362 | | 364 | 365 |
| | | | | | $\bar{x}$ | | | | | 101 | | 95 | 87 | | $\bar{x}$ | | | | | 41 | | 45 | 44 |
| | | | | | $P_{98}$ | | | | | 339 | | 324 | 273 | | $P_{98}$ | | | | | 131 | | 149 | 134 |
| | | | | | max | | | | | 428 | | 396 | 382 | | max | | | | | 262 | | 219 | 194 |
| | | 4 | CCR | Acid | *n* | | | | | | 365 | 364 | 366 | Smoke | *n* | | | | | | 363 | 364 | 334 |
| | | | | | $\bar{x}$ | | | | | | 95 | 84 | 81 | | $\bar{x}$ | | | | | | 52 | 50 | 51 |
| | | | | | $P_{98}$ | | | | | | 305 | 308 | 252 | | $P_{98}$ | | | | | | 171 | 156 | 137 |
| | | | | | max | | | | | | 687 | 417 | 330 | | max | | | | | | 207 | 201 | 199 |

| | | | | | | | | | | | | | | | | | | | | | |
|---|---|---|---|---|---|---|---|---|---|---|---|---|---|---|---|---|---|---|---|---|---|
| France (*cont.*) | Toulouse | 1 | CCI | Acid | *n*<br>x̃<br>$P_{98}$<br>max | | | | | 216<br>6<br>40<br>88 | 209<br>4<br>16<br>87 | 309<br>6<br>35<br>66 | | Smoke | *n*<br>x̃<br>$P_{98}$<br>max | | | | | 331<br>22<br>72<br>133 | 176*<br>23*<br>93*<br>137* | 290<br>26<br>99<br>203 | |
| | | 2 | CCC | Acid | *n*<br>x̃<br>$P_{98}$<br>max | | | | | 303<br>39<br>108<br>153 | 214*<br>42*<br>110*<br>166* | | | Smoke | *n*<br>x̃<br>$P_{98}$<br>max | | | | | 303<br>179<br>450<br>637 | 203*<br>136*<br>407*<br>485* | | |
| | | 3 | CCR | Acid | *n*<br>x̃<br>$P_{98}$<br>max | | | | | 228<br>7<br>34<br>49 | 217<br>5<br>21<br>57 | 301<br>7<br>37<br>48 | | Smoke | *n*<br>x̃<br>$P_{98}$<br>max | | | | | 332<br>15<br>52<br>89 | 215<br>17<br>67<br>95 | 300<br>18<br>65<br>180 | |
| Germany, Federal Republic of | Frankfurt | 1 | SI | Cond | *n*<br>x̃<br>$P_{98}$<br>max | 317<br>86<br>251<br>346 | 302<br>86<br>210<br>390 | 290<br>77<br>245<br>408 | 168*<br>58*<br>119*<br>132* | 158*<br>75*<br>336*<br>390* | 233*<br>58*<br>208*<br>278* | 191*<br>40*<br>75*<br>139* | 166*<br>32*<br>81*<br>104* | | | | | | | | | | |
| | | 2 | CCC | Cond | *n*<br>x̃<br>$P_{98}$<br>max | 321<br>107<br>296<br>407 | 321<br>109<br>246<br>417 | 320<br>98<br>295<br>478 | 314<br>95<br>243<br>354 | 299<br>76<br>202<br>333 | 307<br>81<br>224<br>260 | 323<br>78<br>237<br>362 | 313<br>74<br>196<br>245 | β-abs | *n*<br>x̃<br>$P_{98}$<br>max | 243*<br>33*<br>84*<br>163* | 49<br>60*<br>154*<br>160* | 210*<br>58*<br>178*<br>377* | 161*<br>40*<br>103*<br>162* | 334<br>33<br>76<br>92 | 301<br>30<br>76<br>94 | 196*<br>32*<br>84*<br>94* | 318<br>27<br>67<br>94 |
| | | 3 | CCR | Cond | *n*<br>x̃<br>$P_{98}$<br>max | 193*<br>16*<br>59*<br>97* | 282*<br>30*<br>97*<br>150* | 212*<br>26*<br>104*<br>135* | 197*<br>37*<br>150*<br>220* | | | | | | | | | | | | | | |
| Ghana | Accra | 1 | SR | TCM | *n*<br>x̃<br>$P_{98}$<br>max | | | | | | 16*<br>18*<br>82*<br>82* | | | Hi-vol | *n*<br>x̃<br>$P_{98}$<br>max | | | | | | 16*<br>75*<br>162*<br>162* | | |
| | | 2 | SI | TCM | *n*<br>x̃<br>$P_{98}$<br>max | | | | | | 14*<br>90*<br>815*<br>815* | | | Hi-vol | *n*<br>x̃<br>$P_{98}$<br>max | | | | | | 43*<br>96*<br>175*<br>175* | | |
| | | 3 | CCC | TCM | *n*<br>x̃<br>$P_{98}$<br>max | | | | | | 5*<br>34*<br>99*<br>99* | | | Hi-vol | *n*<br>x̃<br>$P_{98}$<br>max | | | | | | 5*<br>398*<br>480*<br>480* | | |

Annex 4 (*cont.*)

| Country | City | Site No. | Site Area | SO₂ Method | | SO₂ 73 | 74 | 75 | 76 | 77 | 78 | 79 | 80 | SPM Method | | SPM 73 | 74 | 75 | 76 | 77 | 78 | 79 | 80 |
|---|---|---|---|---|---|---|---|---|---|---|---|---|---|---|---|---|---|---|---|---|---|---|---|
| Greece | Athens | 1 | SR | TCM | $n$ | | | | | | 307 | 126 | | Hi-vol | $n$ | | | | | | 101 | 16* | |
| | | | | | $\bar{x}$ | | | | | | 30 | 38* | | | $\bar{x}$ | | | | | | 215 | 235* | |
| | | | | | $P_{98}$ | | | | | | 67 | 100* | | | $P_{98}$ | | | | | | 374 | 462* | |
| | | | | | max | | | | | | 111 | 385* | | | max | | | | | | 536 | 462* | |
| | | 2 | SI | TCM | $n$ | | | | | | 241* | 113* | 181* | Hi-vol | $n$ | | | | | | 90 | 34* | 41* |
| | | | | | $\bar{x}$ | | | | | | 43* | 60* | 49* | | $\bar{x}$ | | | | | | 204 | 245* | 202* |
| | | | | | $P_{98}$ | | | | | | 158* | 232* | 230* | | $P_{98}$ | | | | | | 388 | 503* | 369* |
| | | | | | max | | | | | | 325* | 585* | 380* | | max | | | | | | 409 | 505* | 464* |
| | | 3 | CCC | TCM | $n$ | | | | | | 297 | 243 | 195 | Hi-vol | $n$ | | | | | | 96 | 62* | 57* |
| | | | | | $\bar{x}$ | | | | | | 39 | 57 | 44 | | $\bar{x}$ | | | | | | 255 | 264* | 218* |
| | | | | | $P_{98}$ | | | | | | 109 | 287 | 198 | | $P_{98}$ | | | | | | 421 | 513* | 342* |
| | | | | | max | | | | | | 165 | 485 | 340 | | max | | | | | | 438 | 521* | 369* |
| Hong Kong | Hong Kong | 1 | CCC | Acid | $n$ | | | 357 | 366 | 354 | 357 | 365 | 366 | Smoke | $n$ | | | 353 | 366 | 349 | 356 | 365 | 366 |
| | | | | | $\bar{x}$ | | | 15 | 5 | 13 | 25 | 33 | 45 | | $\bar{x}$ | | | 48 | 53 | 63 | 57 | 46 | 49 |
| | | | | | $P_{98}$ | | | 72 | 34 | 77 | 146 | 99 | 138 | | $P_{98}$ | | | 98 | 117 | 149 | 176 | 97 | 105 |
| | | | | | max | | | 188 | 74 | 152 | 230 | 198 | 290 | | max | | | 112 | 134 | 212 | 281 | 164 | 198 |
| | | 2 | SI | Acid | $n$ | | | 364 | 366 | 364 | 365 | 365 | 366 | Smoke | $n$ | | | 364 | 366 | 364 | 365 | 365 | 366 |
| | | | | | $\bar{x}$ | | | 100 | 44 | 23 | 65 | 58 | 70 | | $\bar{x}$ | | | 28 | 29 | 30 | 30 | 29 | 25 |
| | | | | | $P_{98}$ | | | 621 | 226 | 152 | 549 | 331 | 330 | | $P_{98}$ | | | 77 | 65 | 66 | 81 | 69 | 60 |
| | | | | | max | | | 896 | 630 | 462 | 912 | 565 | 494 | | max | | | 170 | 97 | 90 | 399 | 116 | 102 |
| | | 3 | SR | Acid | $n$ | | | 362 | 366 | 364 | 362 | 365 | 366 | Smoke | $n$ | | | 358 | 366 | 363 | 361 | 365 | 366 |
| | | | | | $\bar{x}$ | | | 20 | 12 | 14 | 30 | 33 | 32 | | $\bar{x}$ | | | 93 | 104 | 120 | 118 | 96 | 91 |
| | | | | | $P_{98}$ | | | 68 | 66 | 98 | 132 | 77 | 90 | | $P_{98}$ | | | 176 | 202 | 265 | 281 | 170 | 175 |
| | | | | | max | | | 132 | 92 | 197 | 553 | 124 | 109 | | max | | | 202 | 269 | 348 | 845 | 227 | 382 |

| | | | | | | | | | | | | | | | | | | | | | | | |
|---|---|---|---|---|---|---|---|---|---|---|---|---|---|---|---|---|---|---|---|---|---|---|---|
| India | Bombay | 1 | CCC | TCM | $n$ | | | | | | 40 | 28 | 29 | Hi-vol | $n$ | | | | | | 40 | 27 | 29 |
| | | | | | $\bar{x}$ | | | | | | 26 | 20 | 21 | | $\bar{x}$ | | | | | | 136 | 179 | 142 |
| | | | | | $P_{98}$ | | | | | | 78 | 83 | 58 | | $P_{98}$ | | | | | | 286 | 314 | 323 |
| | | | | | max | | | | | | 123 | 86 | 59 | | max | | | | | | 381 | 326 | 337 |
| | | 2 | SR | TCM | $n$ | | | | | | 75 | 67 | 26* | Hi-vol | $n$ | | | | | | 75 | 68 | 29* |
| | | | | | $\bar{x}$ | | | | | | 31 | 22 | 26* | | $\bar{x}$ | | | | | | 466 | 174 | 194* |
| | | | | | $P_{98}$ | | | | | | 110 | 61 | 71* | | $P_{98}$ | | | | | | 328 | 313 | 351* |
| | | | | | max | | | | | | 133 | 82 | 88* | | max | | | | | | 334 | 447 | 361* |
| | | 3 | SC | TCM | $n$ | | | | | | 75 | 69 | 27* | Hi-vol | $n$ | | | | | | 69 | 69 | 31* |
| | | | | | $\bar{x}$ | | | | | | 96 | 83 | 48* | | $\bar{x}$ | | | | | | 234 | 275 | 211* |
| | | | | | $P_{98}$ | | | | | | 245 | 203 | 98* | | $P_{98}$ | | | | | | 474 | 551 | 427* |
| | | | | | max | | | | | | 262 | 304 | 112* | | max | | | | | | 518 | 560 | 441* |
| | Calcutta | 1 | CCC | TCM | $n$ | 91 | 58* | 52 | 57 | 40 | 41 | 48 | 31 | Hi-vol | $n$ | 45 | 45 | 23 | 29 | 40 | 41 | 48 | 31 |
| | | | | | $\bar{x}$ | 40 | 62* | 37 | 41 | 47 | 40 | 43 | 48 | | $\bar{x}$ | 365 | 519 | 547 | 356 | 419 | 393 | 439 | 462 |
| | | | | | $P_{98}$ | 221 | 173* | 139 | 135 | 177 | 148 | 152 | 127 | | $P_{98}$ | 651 | 917 | 1038 | 606 | 789 | 730 | 881 | 899 |
| | | | | | max | 244 | 367* | 149 | 161 | 366 | 158 | 227 | 229 | | max | 724 | 1090 | 1038 | 653 | 812 | 751 | 917 | 997 |
| | | 3 | SI | TCM | $n$ | 86 | 54* | 49 | 63 | 35 | 45 | 43 | 30 | Hi-vol | $n$ | 43 | 41 | 22 | 31 | 35 | 45 | 42 | 30 |
| | | | | | $\bar{x}$ | 46 | 68* | 40 | 39 | 58 | 54 | 48 | 48 | | $\bar{x}$ | 330 | 454 | 530 | 380 | 373 | 353 | 413 | 356 |
| | | | | | $P_{98}$ | 156 | 241* | 151 | 170 | 168 | 183 | 201 | 155 | | $P_{98}$ | 893 | 841 | 807 | 640 | 701 | 658 | 845 | 641 |
| | | | | | max | 225 | 282* | 212 | 279 | 223 | 251 | 215 | 196 | | max | 1019 | 1011 | 807 | 680 | 731 | 700 | 897 | 881 |
| | | 4 | SR | TCM | $n$ | 92 | 56* | 52 | 65 | 39 | 40 | 30 | 27 | Hi-vol | $n$ | 44 | 41 | 22 | 33 | 39 | 40 | 30 | 27 |
| | | | | | $\bar{x}$ | 36 | 39* | 28 | 22 | 22 | 20 | 34 | 17 | | $\bar{x}$ | 300 | 365 | 395 | 326 | 354 | 292 | 498 | 394 |
| | | | | | $P_{98}$ | 197 | 142* | 116 | 73 | 82 | 74 | 90 | 69 | | $P_{98}$ | 878 | 699 | 807 | 627 | 775 | 648 | 1044 | 811 |
| | | | | | max | 252 | 160* | 126 | 105 | 95 | 115 | 106 | 74 | | max | 878 | 813 | 807 | 667 | 1763 | 713 | 1111 | 1415 |
| | Delhi | 1 | CCC | TCM | $n$ | | | | | | 44 | 41 | 34 | Hi-vol | $n$ | | | | | | 44 | 42 | 35 |
| | | | | | $\bar{x}$ | | | | | | 34 | 39 | 50 | | $\bar{x}$ | | | | | | 408 | 474 | 535 |
| | | | | | $P_{98}$ | | | | | | 98 | 108 | 121 | | $P_{98}$ | | | | | | 914 | 812 | 1148 |
| | | | | | max | | | | | | 130 | 109 | 135 | | max | | | | | | 980 | 845 | 2221 |
| | | 2 | CCR | TCM | $n$ | | | | | | 33 | 41 | 39 | Hi-vol | $n$ | | | | | | 33 | 41 | 39 |
| | | | | | $\bar{x}$ | | | | | | 8 | 11 | 19 | | $\bar{x}$ | | | | | | 326 | 305 | 322 |
| | | | | | $P_{98}$ | | | | | | 24 | 30 | 71 | | $P_{98}$ | | | | | | 687 | 682 | 590 |
| | | | | | max | | | | | | 67 | 56 | 140 | | max | | | | | | 961 | 751 | 670 |
| | | 3 | CCI | TCM | $n$ | | | | | | 34 | 41 | 40 | Hi-vol | $n$ | | | | | | 34 | 41 | 40 |
| | | | | | $\bar{x}$ | | | | | | 58 | 31 | 47 | | $\bar{x}$ | | | | | | 432 | 440 | 453 |
| | | | | | $P_{98}$ | | | | | | 181 | 122 | 122 | | $P_{98}$ | | | | | | 739 | 830 | 732 |
| | | | | | max | | | | | | 474 | 135 | 151 | | max | | | | | | 972 | 875 | 879 |

Annex 4 (*cont.*)

| Country | City | Site No. | Site Area | SO2 Method | | SO2 73 | SO2 74 | SO2 75 | SO2 76 | SO2 77 | SO2 78 | SO2 79 | SO2 80 | SPM Method | | SPM 73 | SPM 74 | SPM 75 | SPM 76 | SPM 77 | SPM 78 | SPM 79 | SPM 80 |
|---|---|---|---|---|---|---|---|---|---|---|---|---|---|---|---|---|---|---|---|---|---|---|---|
| Indonesia | Jakarta | 1 | CCR | | | | | | | | | | | Hi-vol | $n$ | | | | | | 10* | 53 | 57 |
| | | | | | | | | | | | | | | | $\bar{x}$ | | | | | | 210* | 255 | 275 |
| | | | | | | | | | | | | | | | $P_{98}$ | | | | | | 438* | 463 | 480 |
| | | | | | | | | | | | | | | | max | | | | | | 438* | 654 | 525 |
| | | 2 | SI | | | | | | | | | | | Hi-vol | $n$ | | | | | | 10* | 56 | 50 |
| | | | | | | | | | | | | | | | $\bar{x}$ | | | | | | 129* | 138 | 167 |
| | | | | | | | | | | | | | | | $P_{98}$ | | | | | | 173* | 277 | 395 |
| | | | | | | | | | | | | | | | max | | | | | | 173* | 327 | 517 |
| Iran (Islamic Republic of) | Tehran | 1 | CCC | Acid | $n$ | | | | 70 | 54 | 77 | 70 | 80 | Hi-vol | $n$ | | | | 44 | 51 | 77 | 69 | 80 |
| | | | | | $\bar{x}$ | | | | 84 | 64 | 46 | 48 | 160 | | $\bar{x}$ | | | | 330 | 361 | 362 | 322 | 292 |
| | | | | | $P_{98}$ | | | | 165 | 160 | 115 | 112 | 403 | | $P_{98}$ | | | | 555 | 696 | 551 | 597 | 510 |
| | | | | | max | | | | 267 | 192 | 152 | 179 | 448 | | max | | | | 627 | 858 | 592 | 885 | 663 |
| | | | | | | | | | | | | | | Smoke | $n$ | | | | 69 | 68 | 77 | 70 | 80 |
| | | | | | | | | | | | | | | | $\bar{x}$ | | | | 232 | 206 | 204 | 209 | 175 |
| | | | | | | | | | | | | | | | $P_{98}$ | | | | 458 | 466 | 461 | 495 | 369 |
| | | | | | | | | | | | | | | | max | | | | 459 | 485 | 806 | 798 | 510 |
| | | 2 | SI | Acid | $n$ | | | | 21* | 46* | 71 | 59 | 66 | Hi-vol | $n$ | | | | 19* | 45* | 60 | 50 | 60 |
| | | | | | $\bar{x}$ | | | | 105* | 60* | 40 | 43 | 110 | | $\bar{x}$ | | | | 429* | 491* | 450 | 459 | 370 |
| | | | | | $P_{98}$ | | | | 155* | 115* | 75 | 84 | 327 | | $P_{98}$ | | | | 750* | 873* | 898 | 812 | 603 |
| | | | | | max | | | | 155* | 139* | 155 | 96 | 340 | | max | | | | 750* | 950* | 915 | 864 | 710 |
| | | | | | | | | | | | | | | Smoke | $n$ | | | | 20* | 53* | 72 | 61 | 69 |
| | | | | | | | | | | | | | | | $\bar{x}$ | | | | 263* | 242* | 234 | 244 | 222 |
| | | | | | | | | | | | | | | | $P_{98}$ | | | | 521* | 515* | 445 | 365 | 515 |
| | | | | | | | | | | | | | | | max | | | | 521* | 518* | 510 | 432 | 540 |
| | | 3 | SR | Acid | $n$ | | | | 23* | 42* | 72 | 61 | 76 | Hi-vol | $n$ | | | | 7* | 41* | 74 | 60 | 65 |
| | | | | | $\bar{x}$ | | | | 99* | 72* | 48 | 44 | 140 | | $\bar{x}$ | | | | 229* | 297* | 399 | 285 | 285 |
| | | | | | $P_{98}$ | | | | 237* | 204* | 142 | 138 | 419 | | $P_{98}$ | | | | 323* | 507* | 721 | 606 | 599 |
| | | | | | max | | | | 237* | 215* | 193 | 152 | 484 | | max | | | | 323* | 575* | 927 | 631 | 603 |
| | | | | | | | | | | | | | | Smoke | $n$ | | | | 23* | 48 | 76 | 65 | 76 |
| | | | | | | | | | | | | | | | $\bar{x}$ | | | | 119* | 90 | 120 | 113 | 128 |
| | | | | | | | | | | | | | | | $P_{98}$ | | | | 308* | 257 | 236 | 355 | 392 |
| | | | | | | | | | | | | | | | max | | | | 308* | 277 | 414 | 385 | 449 |

| | | | | | | | | | | | | | | | | | | | | | |
|---|---|---|---|---|---|---|---|---|---|---|---|---|---|---|---|---|---|---|---|---|---|
| Iraq | Baghdad | 1 | SI | TCM | $n$ | | | | | 34* | 86* | 12* | | Hi-vol | $n$ | | | | | 34* | 62* | | |
| | | | | | $\bar{x}$ | | | | | 26* | 17* | 7* | | | $\bar{x}$ | | | | | 362* | 328* | | |
| | | | | | $P_{98}$ | | | | | 66* | 65* | 35* | | | $P_{98}$ | | | | | 1160* | 1087* | | |
| | | | | | max | | | | | 141* | 88* | 35* | | | max | | | | | 1201* | 1635* | | |
| | | 2 | SI | TCM | $n$ | | | | | 33* | 19* | 14* | | Hi-vol | $n$ | | | | | 12* | 12* | 90* | 34* |
| | | | | | $\bar{x}$ | | | | | 26* | 25* | 19* | | | $\bar{x}$ | | | | | 504* | 265* | 554* | 563* |
| | | | | | $P_{98}$ | | | | | 61* | 106* | 81* | | | $P_{98}$ | | | | | 1197* | 398* | 1724* | 1327* |
| | | | | | max | | | | | 87* | 183* | 81* | | | max | | | | | 1197* | 398* | 1901* | 1685* |
| | | 3 | SI | TCM | $n$ | | | | | 34* | 86* | 13* | | Hi-vol | $n$ | | | | | 34* | 141* | 93* | 33* |
| | | | | | $\bar{x}$ | | | | | 15* | 16* | 10* | | | $\bar{x}$ | | | | | 236* | 327* | 580* | 456* |
| | | | | | $P_{98}$ | | | | | 40* | 60* | 29* | | | $P_{98}$ | | | | | 568* | 987* | 1722 | 811* |
| | | | | | max | | | | | 68* | 88* | 29* | | | max | | | | | 1032* | 1770* | 5287* | 1393* |
| Ireland | Dublin | 1 | CCC | Acid | $n$ | | | | | 365 | 363 | 364 | 366 | Smoke | $n$ | | | | | 364 | 364 | 363 | 350 |
| | | | | | $\bar{x}$ | | | | | 38 | 48 | 47 | 56 | | $\bar{x}$ | | | | | 43 | 33 | 30 | 41 |
| | | | | | $P_{98}$ | | | | | 140 | 149 | 137 | 133 | | $P_{98}$ | | | | | 142 | 115 | 111 | 166 |
| | | | | | max | | | | | 293 | 177 | 193 | 202 | | max | | | | | 200 | 177 | 300 | 269 |
| | | 2 | CCI | Acid | $n$ | | | | | 363 | 364 | 363 | 365 | Smoke | $n$ | | | | | 365 | 363 | 362 | 361 |
| | | | | | $\bar{x}$ | | | | | 30 | 43 | 30 | 34 | | $\bar{x}$ | | | | | 42 | 25 | 14 | 14 |
| | | | | | $P_{98}$ | | | | | 105 | 95 | 78 | 81 | | $P_{98}$ | | | | | 117 | 71 | 52 | 50 |
| | | | | | max | | | | | 260 | 119 | 126 | 157 | | max | | | | | 156 | 125 | 85 | 99 |
| | | 3 | SR | Acid | $n$ | | | | | 347 | 365 | 361 | 366 | Smoke | $n$ | | | | | 349 | 365 | 363 | 365 |
| | | | | | $\bar{x}$ | | | | | 22 | 28 | 21 | 23 | | $\bar{x}$ | | | | | 25 | 21 | 15 | 16 |
| | | | | | $P_{98}$ | | | | | 85 | 84 | 79 | 57 | | $P_{98}$ | | | | | 74 | 75 | 65 | 59 |
| | | | | | max | | | | | 198 | 102 | 116 | 113 | | max | | | | | 131 | 166 | 127 | 169 |

Annex 4 (*cont.*)

| Country | City | Site No. | Site Area | SO2 Method | | SO2 73 | SO2 74 | SO2 75 | SO2 76 | SO2 77 | SO2 78 | SO2 79 | SO2 80 | SPM Method | | SPM 73 | SPM 74 | SPM 75 | SPM 76 | SPM 77 | SPM 78 | SPM 79 | SPM 80 |
|---|---|---|---|---|---|---|---|---|---|---|---|---|---|---|---|---|---|---|---|---|---|---|---|
| Italy | Milan | 1 | CCR | Coul | $n$ | | | | | 277 | 285 | 224* | 277 | | | | | | | | | | |
| | | | | | $\bar{x}$ | | | | | 215 | 220 | 354* | 242 | | | | | | | | | | |
| | | | | | $P_{98}$ | | | | | 894 | 902 | 1305* | 939 | | | | | | | | | | |
| | | | | | max | | | | | 1620 | 1180 | 1641* | 1279 | | | | | | | | | | |
| | | 2 | CCC | Coul | $n$ | | | | | 209 | 241 | 198* | 277 | | | | | | | | | | |
| | | | | | $\bar{x}$ | | | | | 185 | 212 | 209* | 167 | | | | | | | | | | |
| | | | | | $P_{98}$ | | | | | 642 | 614 | 619* | 449 | | | | | | | | | | |
| | | | | | max | | | | | 814 | 850 | 861* | 728 | | | | | | | | | | |
| | Rome | 1 | CCI | Coul | $n$ | 285 | 112* | 218* | | | | | | Smoke | $n$ | 285 | 103* | 219* | | | | | |
| | | | | | $\bar{x}$ | 114 | 89* | 78* | | | | | | | $\bar{x}$ | 31 | 46* | 43* | | | | | |
| | | | | | $P_{98}$ | 666 | 375* | 225* | | | | | | | $P_{98}$ | 88 | 162* | 125* | | | | | |
| | | | | | max | 1500 | 525* | 370* | | | | | | | max | 105 | 207* | 200* | | | | | |
| | | 2 | SR | TCM | $n$ | 200* | 6* | 229* | | | | | | Smoke | $n$ | 189* | 6* | 267 | | | | | |
| | | | | | $\bar{x}$ | 23* | 16* | 14* | | | | | | | $\bar{x}$ | 31* | 28* | 22 | | | | | |
| | | | | | $P_{98}$ | 208* | 28* | 40* | | | | | | | $P_{98}$ | 93* | 34* | 58 | | | | | |
| | | | | | max | 413* | 28* | 61* | | | | | | | max | 118* | 34* | 107 | | | | | |
| | | 3 | CCC | TCM | $n$ | 285 | 101* | 219* | | | | | | Smoke | $n$ | 229* | 102* | 218 | | | | | |
| | | | | | $\bar{x}$ | 58 | 108* | 71* | | | | | | | $\bar{x}$ | 53* | 60* | 80 | | | | | |
| | | | | | $P_{98}$ | 370 | 305* | 265* | | | | | | | $P_{98}$ | 123* | 131* | 124 | | | | | |
| | | | | | max | 874 | 600* | 295* | | | | | | | max | 169* | 160* | 528 | | | | | |
| Israel | Tel Aviv | 1 | CCC | Coul | $n$ | 337 | 320 | 344 | 293 | 126* | | 293 | | | | | | | | | | | |
| | | | | | $\bar{x}$ | 29 | 54 | 16 | 32 | 33* | | 53 | | | | | | | | | | | |
| | | | | | $P_{98}$ | 106 | 176 | 58 | 93 | 146* | | 118 | | | | | | | | | | | |
| | | | | | max | 269 | 307 | 95 | 133 | 210* | | 161 | | | | | | | | | | | |
| | | 2 | CCR | Coul | $n$ | 277 | 356 | 346 | 297 | 153* | | | | | | | | | | | | | |
| | | | | | $\bar{x}$ | 28 | 17 | 27 | 29 | 48* | | | | | | | | | | | | | |
| | | | | | $P_{98}$ | 107 | 64 | 92 | 114 | 131* | | | | | | | | | | | | | |
| | | | | | max | 163 | 130 | 162 | 182 | 170* | | | | | | | | | | | | | |
| | | 3 | CCI | Coul | $n$ | 336 | 331 | 267 | 258 | 63* | | | | | | | | | | | | | |
| | | | | | $\bar{x}$ | 20 | 27 | 20 | 16 | 28* | | | | | | | | | | | | | |
| | | | | | $P_{98}$ | 93 | 101 | 77 | 60 | 103* | | | | | | | | | | | | | |
| | | | | | max | 136 | 157 | 112 | 73 | 103* | | | | | | | | | | | | | |

| | | | | | | | | | | | | | | | | | | | | | | | |
|---|---|---|---|---|---|---|---|---|---|---|---|---|---|---|---|---|---|---|---|---|---|---|---|
| Japan | Osaka | 1 | CCC | Cond | $n$<br>$\bar{x}$<br>$P_{98}$<br>max | | | 273<br>73<br>165<br>191 | 342<br>74<br>141<br>189 | 365<br>70<br>134<br>157 | 363<br>49<br>121<br>136 | 352<br>45<br>86<br>113 | 359<br>34<br>68<br>79 | Neph | $n$<br>$\bar{x}$<br>$P_{98}$<br>max | | | 326<br>81<br>192<br>252 | 294<br>82<br>193<br>459 | 365<br>66<br>138<br>161 | 364<br>53<br>133<br>169 | 361<br>55<br>173<br>230 | 361<br>49<br>119<br>198 |
| | | 2 | CCI | Cond | $n$<br>$\bar{x}$<br>$P_{98}$<br>max | | | 365<br>74<br>131<br>168 | 366<br>66<br>138<br>173 | 359<br>47<br>107<br>147 | 359<br>36<br>97<br>123 | 359<br>37<br>86<br>113 | 358<br>33<br>71<br>89 | Neph | $n$<br>$\bar{x}$<br>$P_{98}$<br>max | | | 365<br>62<br>151<br>220 | 366<br>67<br>140<br>233 | 356<br>59<br>138<br>187 | 361<br>58<br>167<br>237 | 356<br>67<br>212<br>283 | 362<br>60<br>139<br>225 |
| | | 3 | SR | Cond | $n$<br>$\bar{x}$<br>$P_{98}$<br>max | | | 330<br>63<br>118<br>141 | 351<br>56<br>115<br>128 | 355<br>58<br>110<br>162 | 365<br>49<br>86<br>115 | 364<br>39<br>81<br>115 | 366<br>29<br>63<br>71 | Neph | $n$<br>$x$<br>$P_{98}$<br>max | | | 343<br>70<br>169<br>241 | 362<br>81<br>180<br>231 | 365<br>69<br>176<br>235 | 362<br>59<br>159<br>216 | 363<br>67<br>217<br>314 | 362<br>58<br>150<br>267 |
| | | 4 | CCI | Cond | $n$<br>$\bar{x}$<br>$P_{98}$<br>max | | | 362<br>62<br>131<br>199 | 343<br>54<br>118<br>155 | | 352<br>42<br>102<br>126 | 353<br>47<br>100<br>128 | 366<br>41<br>84<br>94 | Neph | $n$<br>$\bar{x}$<br>$P_{98}$<br>max | | | 344<br>85<br>202<br>358 | 364<br>97<br>217<br>317 | | 365<br>53<br>126<br>158 | 362<br>59<br>158<br>272 | 364<br>53<br>133<br>198 |
| | Tokyo | 1 | CCC | Cond | $n$<br>$\bar{x}$<br>$P_{98}$<br>max | 363<br>71<br>140<br>149 | 363<br>68<br>118<br>152 | 363<br>65<br>124<br>186 | 366<br>66<br>118<br>260 | 358<br>68<br>110<br>144 | 364<br>54<br>100<br>123 | 363<br>56<br>102<br>183 | 355<br>55<br>97<br>126 | Neph | $n$<br>$\bar{x}$<br>$P_{98}$<br>max | 67 | 48 | 55 | 366<br>70<br>200<br>229 | 365<br>55<br>178<br>323 | 353<br>59<br>185<br>272 | 365<br>63<br>205<br>337 | 354<br>59<br>191<br>312 |
| | | 2 | SR | Cond | $n$<br>$\bar{x}$<br>$P_{98}$<br>max | 359<br>48<br>106<br>133 | 346<br>43<br>93<br>112 | 361<br>49<br>104<br>134 | 365<br>52<br>110<br>160 | 365<br>47<br>73<br>100 | 365<br>45<br>86<br>100 | 365<br>46<br>76<br>105 | 361<br>37<br>68<br>81 | Neph | $n$<br>$\bar{x}$<br>$P_{98}$<br>max | 72 | 67 | 61 | 313<br>68<br>182<br>221 | 365<br>57<br>175<br>294 | 365<br>52<br>167<br>281 | 364<br>57<br>190<br>282 | 315<br>52<br>181<br>268 |
| | | 3 | CCI | Cond | $n$<br>$\bar{x}$<br>$P_{98}$<br>max | 365<br>77<br>155<br>195 | 358<br>85<br>145<br>312 | 364<br>71<br>130<br>175 | 366<br>80<br>157<br>244 | 365<br>79<br>128<br>181 | 365<br>62<br>131<br>207 | 352<br>68<br>136<br>178 | 361<br>59<br>102<br>121 | Neph | $n$<br>$\bar{x}$<br>$P_{98}$<br>max | 77 | 64 | 60 | 366<br>73<br>180<br>245 | 365<br>60<br>173<br>309 | 365<br>59<br>178<br>291 | 364<br>59<br>195<br>263 | 361<br>56<br>161<br>294 |
| Kenya | Nairobi | 1 | CCR | TCM | $n$<br>$\bar{x}$<br>$P_{98}$<br>max | | | | | 5*<br>16*<br>25*<br>25* | 8*<br>49*<br>61*<br>62* | | | Hi-vol | $n$<br>$\bar{x}$<br>$P_{98}$<br>max | | | | | 6*<br>71*<br>88*<br>88* | 8*<br>89*<br>128*<br>128* | | |
| | | 2 | SI | TCM | $n$<br>$\bar{x}$<br>$P_{98}$<br>max | | | | | 6*<br>36*<br>51*<br>51* | 6*<br>56*<br>142*<br>142* | | | Hi-vol | $n$<br>$\bar{x}$<br>$P_{98}$<br>max | | | | | 6*<br>51*<br>60*<br>60* | 12*<br>80*<br>124*<br>124* | | |

Annex 4 (*cont.*)

| Country | City | Site | | SO$_2$ | | | | | | | | | | SPM | | | | | | | | | |
|---|---|---|---|---|---|---|---|---|---|---|---|---|---|---|---|---|---|---|---|---|---|---|---|
| | | | | | | Year | | | | | | | | | | Year | | | | | | | |
| | | No. | Area | Method | | 73 | 74 | 75 | 76 | 77 | 78 | 79 | 80 | Method | | 73 | 74 | 75 | 76 | 77 | 78 | 79 | 80 |
| Malaysia | Kuala Lumpur | 1 | SI | TCM | *n* | | | | | | 140 | 125 | 118 | Hi-vol | *n* | | | | | | 114 | 125 | 137 |
| | | | | | $\bar{x}$ | | | | | | 43 | 15 | 22 | | $\bar{x}$ | | | | | | 153 | 158 | 182 |
| | | | | | $P_{98}$ | | | | | | 91 | 51 | 108 | | $P_{98}$ | | | | | | 246 | 293 | 329 |
| | | | | | max | | | | | | 101 | 63 | 116 | | max | | | | | | 275 | 498 | 464 |
| | | 2 | SR | TCM | *n* | | | | | | 140 | 102 | 45* | Hi-vol | *n* | | | | | | 130 | 121 | 110 |
| | | | | | $\bar{x}$ | | | | | | 5 | 3 | 3* | | $\bar{x}$ | | | | | | 90 | 79 | 98 |
| | | | | | $P_{98}$ | | | | | | 19 | 5 | 5* | | $P_{98}$ | | | | | | 160 | 124 | 249 |
| | | | | | max | | | | | | 20 | 16 | 9 | | max | | | | | | 203 | 182 | 298 |
| Netherlands | Amsterdam | 1 | CCC | Coul | *n* | 307 | 343 | 341 | 345 | 314* | 294* | 352 | 338 | | | | | | | | | | |
| | | | | | $\bar{x}$ | 55 | 30 | 44 | 36 | 29* | 32* | 42 | 26 | | | | | | | | | | |
| | | | | | $P_{98}$ | 196 | 78 | 176 | 144 | 94* | 118* | 195 | 66 | | | | | | | | | | |
| | | | | | max | 319 | 156 | 321 | 207 | 132* | 162* | 287 | 123 | | | | | | | | | | |
| | | 2 | SR | Coul | *n* | 312 | 354 | 350 | 340 | 354 | 308* | 343 | 357 | | | | | | | | | | |
| | | | | | $\bar{x}$ | 39 | 23 | 25 | 27 | 21 | 26* | 41 | 30 | | | | | | | | | | |
| | | | | | $P_{98}$ | 151 | 72 | 86 | 92 | 67 | 103* | 172 | 98 | | | | | | | | | | |
| | | | | | max | 212 | 110 | 128 | 166 | 111 | 131* | 305 | 215 | | | | | | | | | | |
| | | 3 | SI | Coul | *n* | 310 | 345 | 352 | 342 | 341 | 313 | 332 | 351 | | | | | | | | | | |
| | | | | | $\bar{x}$ | 53 | 35 | 38 | 33 | 32 | 32 | 30 | 28 | | | | | | | | | | |
| | | | | | $P_{98}$ | 179 | 117 | 140 | 122 | 98 | 114 | 168 | 80 | | | | | | | | | | |
| | | | | | max | 317 | 192 | 168 | 252 | 134 | 145 | 273 | 165 | | | | | | | | | | |

| | | | | | | | | | | | | | | | | | | | | | |
|---|---|---|---|---|---|---|---|---|---|---|---|---|---|---|---|---|---|---|---|---|---|
| New Zealand | Auckland | 1 | SI | Acid | $n$<br>$\bar{x}$<br>$P_{98}$<br>max | | | 78*<br>20*<br>50*<br>66* | 142*<br>20*<br>47*<br>58* | 356<br>20<br>43<br>53 | 310<br>25<br>61<br>108 | 349<br>22<br>45<br>65 | 341<br>25<br>50<br>74 | Smoke | $n$<br>$\bar{x}$<br>$P_{98}$<br>max | | | 96*<br>6*<br>18*<br>21* | 145*<br>5*<br>14*<br>19* | 354<br>9<br>35<br>62 | 309<br>6<br>22<br>50 | 340<br>5<br>19<br>47 | 831<br>6<br>21<br>41 |
| | | 2 | CCC | Acid | $n$<br>$\bar{x}$<br>$P_{98}$<br>max | | | 280*<br>18*<br>29*<br>37* | 345<br>12<br>33<br>47 | 355<br>12<br>26<br>39 | 303<br>25<br>108<br>165 | 330<br>15<br>32<br>55 | 358<br>15<br>31<br>38 | Smoke | $n$<br>$\bar{x}$<br>$P_{98}$<br>max | | | 279*<br>5*<br>26*<br>38* | 335<br>4<br>15<br>24 | 350<br>4<br>18<br>37 | 333<br>4<br>14<br>26 | 321<br>4<br>18<br>32 | 349<br>5<br>20<br>30 |
| | | 3 | CCR | Acid | $n$<br>$\bar{x}$<br>$P_{98}$<br>max | | | | | | 331<br>19<br>76<br>165 | 332<br>15<br>33<br>42 | 359<br>11<br>25<br>56 | Smoke | $n$<br>$\bar{x}$<br>$P_{98}$<br>max | | | | | | 337<br>4<br>21<br>45 | 349<br>5<br>29<br>42 | 360<br>6<br>30<br>38 |
| | Christ-church | 1 | SR | Acid | $n$<br>$\bar{x}$<br>$P_{98}$<br>max | | | | 84*<br>42*<br>105*<br>156* | 235*<br>18*<br>63*<br>232* | 323<br>17<br>45<br>72 | 330<br>20<br>58<br>81 | 323<br>23<br>61<br>87 | Smoke | $n$<br>$\bar{x}$<br>$P_{98}$<br>max | | | | 112*<br>67*<br>304*<br>516* | 241*<br>34*<br>195*<br>253* | 353<br>26<br>187<br>332 | 358<br>31<br>215<br>497 | 325<br>41<br>280<br>538 |
| | | 2 | SI | Acid | $n$<br>$\bar{x}$<br>$P_{98}$<br>max | | | | | | 259<br>23<br>72<br>94 | 304<br>32<br>85<br>145 | 349<br>37<br>84<br>107 | Smoke | $n$<br>$\bar{x}$<br>$P_{98}$<br>max | | | | | | 266*<br>19*<br>138*<br>245* | 308<br>19<br>127<br>336 | 354<br>21<br>155<br>332 |
| | | 3 | SC | Acid | $n$<br>$\bar{x}$<br>$P_{98}$<br>max | | | | | | 337<br>26<br>68<br>135 | 335<br>31<br>81<br>106 | 316<br>34<br>73<br>94 | Smoke | $n$<br>$\bar{x}$<br>$P_{98}$<br>max | | | | | | 339<br>20<br>151<br>274 | 329<br>29<br>205<br>314 | 316<br>32<br>199<br>417 |
| Pakistan | Lahore | 1 | SR | TCM | $n$<br>$\bar{x}$<br>$P_{98}$<br>max | | | | | | | 29*<br>40*<br>62*<br>68* | | Hi-vol | $n$<br>$\bar{x}$<br>$P_{98}$<br>max | | | | | | | 69*<br>749*<br>2740*<br>3415* | 106*<br>690*<br>1391*<br>1682* |
| | | 2 | CCC | TCM | $n$<br>$\bar{x}$<br>$P_{98}$<br>max | | | | | | 99*<br>49*<br>63*<br>65* | | | Hi-vol | $n$<br>$\bar{x}$<br>$P_{98}$<br>max | | | | | | 99*<br>332*<br>618*<br>667* | | |

Annex 4 (*cont.*)

| Country | City | Site No. | Site Area | $SO_2$ Method | | $SO_2$ 73 | 74 | 75 | 76 | 77 | 78 | 79 | 80 | SPM Method | | SPM 73 | 74 | 75 | 76 | 77 | 78 | 79 | 80 |
|---|---|---|---|---|---|---|---|---|---|---|---|---|---|---|---|---|---|---|---|---|---|---|---|
| Peru | Lima | 1 | CCC | Acid | $n$ | | | | 103* | | | 127 | 36* | Smoke | $n$ | | | | 90* | | | 144 | 68* |
| | | | | | $\bar{x}$ | | | | 15* | | | 3 | 6* | | $\bar{x}$ | | | | 33* | | | 6 | 10* |
| | | | | | $P_{98}$ | | | | 31* | | | 10 | 21* | | $P_{98}$ | | | | 75* | | | 28 | 49* |
| | | | | | max | | | | 105* | | | 11 | 27* | | max | | | | 113* | | | 34 | 64* |
| | | 2 | CCR | Acid | $n$ | | | | 185 | 46* | 121* | 118* | 67* | Smoke | $n$ | | | | 263 | 39* | 77* | 118* | 67* |
| | | | | | $\bar{x}$ | | | | 11 | 9* | 14* | 4* | 7* | | $\bar{x}$ | | | | 26 | 13* | 12* | 5* | 14* |
| | | | | | $P_{98}$ | | | | 22 | 17* | 38* | 25* | 25* | | $P_{98}$ | | | | 73 | 19* | 18* | 30* | 41* |
| | | | | | max | | | | 47 | 19* | 43* | 33* | 43* | | max | | | | 101 | 20* | 27* | 31* | 58* |
| | | 3 | SR | Acid | $n$ | | | | 23* | | | | 34* | Smoke | $n$ | | | | 132* | 37* | 71 | 59* | 34* |
| | | | | | $\bar{x}$ | | | | 6* | | | | 8* | | $\bar{x}$ | | | | 31* | 24* | 21 | 25* | 31* |
| | | | | | $P_{98}$ | | | | 51* | | | | 38* | | $P_{98}$ | | | | 54* | 47* | 34 | 42* | 58* |
| | | | | | max | | | | 51* | | | | 38* | | max | | | | 73* | 50* | 39 | 49* | 58* |
| Philippines | Iligan City | 2 | SI | | | | | | | | | | | Hi-vol | $n$ | | | | | | | 27* | 29* |
| | | | | | | | | | | | | | | | $\bar{x}$ | | | | | | | 208* | 173* |
| | | | | | | | | | | | | | | | $P_{98}$ | | | | | | | 332* | 192* |
| | | | | | | | | | | | | | | | max | | | | | | | 335* | 392* |
| | Manila | 1 | SR | Cond | $n$ | | | 348 | 349 | 361 | 354 | 272 | 251 | Neph | $n$ | | | 341 | 346 | 361 | 356 | 257 | 219 |
| | | | | | $\bar{x}$ | | | 67 | 55 | 54 | 46 | 58 | 62 | | $\bar{x}$ | | | 71 | 76 | 93 | 87 | 101 | 99 |
| | | | | | $P_{98}$ | | | 139 | 94 | 102 | 84 | 115 | 149 | | $P_{98}$ | | | 156 | 135 | 225 | 159 | 188 | 171 |
| | | | | | max | | | 196 | 107 | 121 | 113 | 126 | 191 | | max | | | 218 | 170 | 290 | 280 | 210 | 258 |
| | | 2 | CCC | Cond | $n$ | | | 353 | 291 | 136* | 291 | 139* | 183* | Neph | $n$ | | | 354 | 345 | 291 | 319 | 331 | 271 |
| | | | | | $\bar{x}$ | | | 89 | 77 | 57* | 66 | 91* | 75* | | $\bar{x}$ | | | 77 | 74 | 92 | 87 | 73 | 79 |
| | | | | | $P_{98}$ | | | 178 | 183 | 173* | 144 | 178* | 131 | | $P_{98}$ | | | 128 | 135 | 165 | 122 | 114 | 180 |
| | | | | | max | | | 207 | 223 | 191* | 160 | 223* | 178 | | max | | | 195 | 165 | 252 | 411 | 202 | 286 |
| | | 3 | SI | Cond | $n$ | | | 360 | 330 | 307 | 173* | 146* | 169* | Neph | $n$ | | | 358 | 337 | 305 | 218* | 191* | 176* |
| | | | | | $\bar{x}$ | | | 130 | 81 | 82 | 91* | 100* | 79 | | $\bar{x}$ | | | 90 | 86 | 94 | 76* | 82* | 92* |
| | | | | | $P_{98}$ | | | 249 | 157 | 178 | 202* | 189* | 176 | | 98 | | | 167 | 160 | 163 | 134* | 119* | 141* |
| | | | | | max | | | 278 | 204 | 265 | 288* | 244* | 249 | | max | | | 211 | 211 | 192 | 165* | 149* | 177* |

| | | | | | | | | | | | | | | | | | | | | | |
|---|---|---|---|---|---|---|---|---|---|---|---|---|---|---|---|---|---|---|---|---|---|
| Poland | Warsaw | 1 | CCR | TCM | *n*<br>x̄<br>$P_{98}$<br>max | | | | | | 161<br>28<br>140<br>180 | 160<br>34<br>160<br>432 | 192<br>35<br>140<br>375 | Smoke | *n*<br>x̄<br>$P_{98}$<br>max | | | | | | 163<br>64<br>195<br>268 | 157<br>40<br>160<br>817 | 188<br>44<br>197<br>481 |
| | | 2 | CCI | TCM | *n*<br>x̄<br>$P_{98}$<br>max | | | | | | 155*<br>38*<br>156*<br>410* | 203<br>43<br>152<br>210 | 208<br>42<br>167<br>269 | Smoke | *n*<br>x̄<br>$P_{98}$<br>max | | | | | | 158*<br>51*<br>140*<br>297* | 190<br>55<br>200<br>414* | 205<br>47<br>281<br>362 |
| | | 3 | CCC | TCM | *n*<br>x̄<br>$P_{98}$<br>max | | | | | | 158*<br>43*<br>170*<br>294* | 213<br>41<br>190<br>262 | 198<br>47<br>202<br>348 | Smoke | *n*<br>x̄<br>$P_{98}$<br>max | | | | | | 159*<br>59*<br>185*<br>359* | 212<br>50<br>170<br>350 | 193<br>56<br>257<br>307 |
| | Wroclaw | 1 | CCC | TCM | *n*<br>x̄<br>$P_{98}$<br>max | | | | | | 291<br>45<br>150<br>200 | 297<br>46<br>169<br>236 | 295<br>45<br>191<br>257 | Smoke | *n*<br>x̄<br>$P_{98}$<br>max | | | | | | 284<br>92<br>302<br>367 | 298<br>77<br>310<br>475 | 293<br>76<br>336<br>570 |
| | | 2 | CCI | TCM | *n*<br>x̄<br>$P_{98}$<br>max | | | | | | 280<br>30<br>110<br>180 | 295<br>34<br>125<br>361 | 291<br>32<br>156<br>237 | Smoke | *n*<br>x̄<br>$P_{98}$<br>max | | | | | | 280<br>64<br>180<br>303 | 291<br>56<br>192<br>225 | 291<br>53<br>176<br>285 |
| | | 3 | CCR | TCM | *n*<br>x̄<br>$P_{98}$<br>max | | | | | | 263<br>23<br>80<br>120 | 292<br>35<br>117<br>160 | 288<br>40<br>189<br>373 | Smoke | *n*<br>x̄<br>$P_{98}$<br>max | | | | | | 261<br>49<br>140<br>190 | 289<br>50<br>146<br>249 | 291<br>52<br>160<br>285 |
| Portugal | Lisbon | 2 | CCR | TCM | *n*<br>x̄<br>$P_{98}$<br>max | | | | | | | | 41*<br>44*<br>105*<br>170* | | | | | | | | | | |
| | | 3 | CCR | TCM | *n*<br>x̄<br>$P_{98}$<br>max | | | | | | | | 163*<br>65*<br>195*<br>270* | | | | | | | | | | |

Annex 4 (*cont.*)

| Country | City | Site | | SO2 | | | | | | | | | | SPM | | | | | | | | | |
|---|---|---|---|---|---|---|---|---|---|---|---|---|---|---|---|---|---|---|---|---|---|---|---|
| | | | | | | Year | | | | | | | | | | Year | | | | | | | |
| | | No. | Area | Method | | 73 | 74 | 75 | 76 | 77 | 78 | 79 | 80 | Method | | 73 | 74 | 75 | 76 | 77 | 78 | 79 | 80 |
| Republic of Korea | Seoul | 1 | CCR | Acid | $n$ | | | | 187* | 180* | | | | | | | | | | | | | |
| | | | | | $\bar{x}$ | | | | 198* | 143* | | | | | | | | | | | | | |
| | | | | | $P_{98}$ | | | | 663* | 403* | | | | | | | | | | | | | |
| | | | | | max | | | | 863* | 511* | | | | | | | | | | | | | |
| | | 2 | SC | Acid | $n$ | | | | 189* | 242* | | | | | | | | | | | | | |
| | | | | | $\bar{x}$ | | | | 144* | 171* | | | | | | | | | | | | | |
| | | | | | $P_{98}$ | | | | 363* | 403* | | | | | | | | | | | | | |
| | | | | | max | | | | 437* | 509* | | | | | | | | | | | | | |
| | | 3 | SI | Acid | $n$ | | | | 172* | 213* | | | | | | | | | | | | | |
| | | | | | $\bar{x}$ | | | | 338* | 315* | | | | | | | | | | | | | |
| | | | | | $P_{98}$ | | | | 840* | 731* | | | | | | | | | | | | | |
| | | | | | max | | | | 966* | 1189* | | | | | | | | | | | | | |
| Spain | Madrid | 1 | CCC | Acid | $n$ | 290 | 303 | 285 | 139* | | 101* | 268 | 281 | Smoke | $n$ | 323 | 300 | 280 | 139* | | 101* | 268 | 281 |
| | | | | | $\bar{x}$ | 168 | 161 | 138 | 136* | | 58* | 102 | 63 | | $\bar{x}$ | 186 | 190 | 211 | 273* | | 108* | 176 | 130 |
| | | | | | $P_{98}$ | 459 | 451 | 399 | 468* | | 118* | 354 | 227 | | $P_{98}$ | 569 | 661 | 618 | 913* | | 247* | 621 | 312 |
| | | | | | max | 606 | 763 | 834 | 499* | | 123* | 605 | 303 | | max | 909 | 908 | 910 | 1080* | | 293* | 821 | 395 |
| | | 2 | SR | Acid | $n$ | 318 | 319 | 316 | 322 | 323 | 180* | 302 | 330 | Smoke | $n$ | 331 | 320 | 315 | 320 | 135* | 180* | 299 | 330 |
| | | | | | $\bar{x}$ | 73 | 63 | 61 | 54 | 44 | 45* | 46 | 30 | | $\bar{x}$ | 72 | 66 | 63 | 67 | 52* | 34* | 66 | 56 |
| | | | | | $P_{98}$ | 227 | 252 | 183 | 144 | 115 | 135* | 168 | 135 | | $P_{98}$ | 264 | 283 | 223 | 288 | 172* | 125* | 289 | 220 |
| | | | | | max | 316 | 296 | 362 | 176 | 134 | 192* | 293 | 163 | | max | 446 | 359 | 297 | 431 | 211* | 156* | 397 | 310 |
| | | 4 | CCI | Acid | $n$ | 320 | 307 | 271 | 294 | 207* | 142* | 253 | | Smoke | $n$ | 322 | 307 | 263 | 294 | 199* | 139* | 252 | |
| | | | | | $\bar{x}$ | 193 | 178 | 133 | 112 | 71* | 78* | 86 | | | $\bar{x}$ | 304 | 307 | 236 | 233 | 157* | 135* | 196 | |
| | | | | | $P_{98}$ | 556 | 556 | 458 | 449 | 173* | 215* | 388 | | | $P_{98}$ | 881 | 958 | 823 | 832 | 401* | 299* | 676 | |
| | | | | | max | 739 | 620 | 829 | 526 | 215* | 332* | 651 | | | max | 1164 | 1312 | 1063 | 1270 | 631* | 591* | 860* | |

| | | | | | | | | | | | | | | | | | | | | | | | |
|---|---|---|---|---|---|---|---|---|---|---|---|---|---|---|---|---|---|---|---|---|---|---|---|
| Sweden | Stockholm | 1 | CCC | Coul | $n$ | | | | 152* | 293 | 295 | 293 | 119* | | | | | | | | | | |
| | | | | | $\bar{x}$ | | | | 63* | 60 | 49 | 58 | 70* | | | | | | | | | | |
| | | | | | $P_{98}$ | | | | 157* | 146 | 139 | 186 | 144* | | | | | | | | | | |
| | | | | | max | | | | 233* | 239 | 200 | 395 | 227* | | | | | | | | | | |
| | | 2 | SR | Coul | $n$ | | | | 149* | 268 | 270 | 314 | 123* | | | | | | | | | | |
| | | | | | $\bar{x}$ | | | | 16* | 17 | 19 | 16 | 19* | | | | | | | | | | |
| | | | | | $P_{98}$ | | | | 50* | 52 | 61 | 55 | 51* | | | | | | | | | | |
| | | | | | max | | | | 105* | 262 | 93 | 91 | 60* | | | | | | | | | | |
| | | 3 | CCC | Coul | $n$ | | | | 58* | 162* | 287 | 313 | 48* | | | | | | | | | | |
| | | | | | $\bar{x}$ | | | | 35* | 44* | 44 | 56 | 44* | | | | | | | | | | |
| | | | | | $P_{98}$ | | | | 84* | 108* | 162 | 202 | 118* | | | | | | | | | | |
| | | | | | max | | | | 88* | 180* | 501 | 284 | 168* | | | | | | | | | | |
| | | 4 | SI | Coul | $n$ | | | | 152* | 261 | 212* | 257 | 117* | | | | | | | | | | |
| | | | | | $\bar{x}$ | | | | 28* | 30 | 50* | 39 | 48* | | | | | | | | | | |
| | | | | | $P_{98}$ | | | | 80* | 114 | 170* | 180 | 164* | | | | | | | | | | |
| | | | | | max | | | | 145* | 146 | 214* | 283 | 185* | | | | | | | | | | |
| | | 5 | CCI | Coul | $n$ | | | | 151* | 271 | 187* | 300 | 88* | | | | | | | | | | |
| | | | | | $\bar{x}$ | | | | 19* | 26 | 23* | 23 | 22* | | | | | | | | | | |
| | | | | | $P_{98}$ | | | | 55* | 79 | 73* | 78 | 58* | | | | | | | | | | |
| | | | | | max | | | | 76* | 122 | 109* | 127 | 80* | | | | | | | | | | |
| Switzer-land | Zürich | 1 | CCC | Cond | $n$ | | | | | 92* | 181* | | | | | | | | | | | | |
| | | | | | $\bar{x}$ | | | | | 78* | 77* | | | | | | | | | | | | |
| | | | | | $P_{98}$ | | | | | 218* | 211* | | | | | | | | | | | | |
| | | | | | max | | | | | 239* | 345* | | | | | | | | | | | | |
| | | | | Acid | $n$ | | | | | | 184* | | | | | | | | | | | | |
| | | | | | $\bar{x}$ | | | | | | 64* | | | | | | | | | | | | |
| | | | | | $P_{98}$ | | | | | | 216* | | | | | | | | | | | | |
| | | | | | max | | | | | | 259* | | | | | | | | | | | | |

Annex 4 (*cont.*)

| Country | City | Site | | $SO_2$ | | | | | | | | | | SPM | | | | | | | | | |
|---|---|---|---|---|---|---|---|---|---|---|---|---|---|---|---|---|---|---|---|---|---|---|---|
| | | | | | | Year | | | | | | | | | | Year | | | | | | | |
| | | No. | Area | Method | | 73 | 74 | 75 | 76 | 77 | 78 | 79 | 80 | Method | | 73 | 74 | 75 | 76 | 77 | 78 | 79 | 80 |
| Thailand | Bangkok | 1 | SI | TCM | *n* | | | | | | 52* | 81* | | Hi-vol | *n* | | | | | | 76 | 120 | 67* |
| | | | | | x̄ | | | | | | 15* | 9* | | | x̄ | | | | | | 162 | 167 | 170 |
| | | | | | $P_{98}$ | | | | | | 50* | 30* | | | $P_{98}$ | | | | | | 330 | 344 | 390 |
| | | | | | max | | | | | | 67* | 37* | | | max | | | | | | 407 | 407 | 413 |
| | | 2 | SR | | | | | | | | | | | Hi-vol | *n* | | | | | | 24* | 75 | 47* |
| | | | | | | | | | | | | | | | x̄ | | | | | | 145* | 176 | 108* |
| | | | | | | | | | | | | | | | $P_{98}$ | | | | | | 237* | 322 | 318* |
| | | | | | | | | | | | | | | | max | | | | | | 237* | 350 | 386* |
| | | 3 | SR | TCM | *n* | | | | | | | 55* | | Hi-vol | *n* | | | | | | 27* | 112 | 11* |
| | | | | | x̄ | | | | | | | 10* | | | x̄ | | | | | | 137* | 170 | 232* |
| | | | | | $P_{98}$ | | | | | | | 37* | | | $P_{98}$ | | | | | | 237* | 302 | 399* |
| | | | | | max | | | | | | | 51* | | | max | | | | | | 286* | 762 | 399* |
| United Kingdom | Glasgow | 1 | CCC | Acid | *n* | | | | | 365 | | 359 | | Smoke | *n* | | | | | 334 | | 365 | |
| | | | | | x̄ | | | | | 94 | | 84 | | | x̄ | | | | | 42 | | 36 | |
| | | | | | $P_{98}$ | | | | | 311 | | 210 | | | $P_{98}$ | | | | | 241 | | 172 | |
| | | | | | max | | | | | 787 | | 409 | | | max | | | | | 529 | | 365 | |
| | | 2 | SR | Acid | *n* | | | | | 351 | 353 | 164 | | Smoke | *n* | | | | | 351 | 353 | 365 | |
| | | | | | x̄ | | | | | 87 | 59 | 44 | | | x̄ | | | | | 21 | 20 | 21 | |
| | | | | | $P_{98}$ | | | | | 172 | 163 | 148 | | | $P_{98}$ | | | | | 184 | 104 | 131 | |
| | | | | | max | | | | | 243 | 437 | 300 | | | max | | | | | 289 | 293 | 253 | |
| | | 3 | CCI | Acid | *n* | | | | | 357 | 365 | 364 | | Smoke | *n* | | | | | 357 | 365 | 364 | |
| | | | | | x̄ | | | | | 86 | 84 | 69 | | | x̄ | | | | | 35 | 28 | 33 | |
| | | | | | $P_{98}$ | | | | | 243 | 208 | 199 | | | $P_{98}$ | | | | | 232 | 133 | 224 | |
| | | | | | max | | | | | 897 | 332 | 367 | | | max | | | | | 471 | 248 | 328 | |
| | London | 1 | CCC | Acid | *n* | 220* | 335 | 363 | 366 | 361 | 365 | 365 | | Smoke | *n* | 221* | 337 | 363 | 366 | 361 | 365 | 365 | |
| | | | | | x̄ | 175* | 137 | 149 | 142 | 86 | 95 | 91 | | | x̄ | 42* | 26 | 35 | 31 | 23 | 21 | 20 | |
| | | | | | $P_{98}$ | 516* | 328 | 515 | 373 | 261 | 302 | 284 | | | $P_{98}$ | 167* | 74 | 124 | 97 | 61 | 63 | 69 | |
| | | | | | max | 798* | 461 | 840 | 636 | 412 | 442 | 569 | | | max | 249* | 149 | 430 | 129 | 111 | 105 | 102 | |
| | | 2 | SR | Acid | *n* | 198 | 213 | 194 | 199 | 210 | 293 | 340 | | Smoke | *n* | 198 | 213 | 194 | 199 | 210 | 297 | 340 | |
| | | | | | x̄ | 102 | 73 | 80 | 84 | 75 | 77 | 77 | | | x̄ | 37 | 26 | 35 | 33 | 26 | 27 | 25 | |
| | | | | | $P_{98}$ | 307 | 211 | 234 | 224 | 203 | 213 | 193 | | | $P_{98}$ | 132 | 92 | 123 | 103 | 78 | 100 | 95 | |
| | | | | | max | 389 | 311 | 621 | 345 | 443 | 270 | 237 | | | max | 218 | 116 | 305 | 229 | 215 | 236 | 205 | |
| | | 3 | SI | Acid | *n* | 162* | 175 | 164 | 139 | 140* | 331 | 330 | | Smoke | *n* | 181 | 175 | 164 | 139 | 140* | 335 | 330 | |
| | | | | | x̄ | 172* | 117 | 65 | 81 | 75* | 56 | 76 | | | x̄ | 48 | 30 | 44 | 27 | 43* | 35 | 84 | |
| | | | | | $P_{98}$ | 359* | 242 | 222 | 181 | 148* | 149 | 127 | | | $P_{98}$ | 184 | 114 | 116 | 82 | 116* | 116 | 171 | |
| | | | | | max | 463* | 304 | 248 | 267 | 157* | 307 | 136 | | | max | 300 | 164 | 134 | 205 | 211* | 248 | 296 | |

| | | | | | | | | | | | | | | | | | | | | | | | |
|---|---|---|---|---|---|---|---|---|---|---|---|---|---|---|---|---|---|---|---|---|---|---|---|
| United States of America | Birmingham, AL | 5 | CCI | TCM | $n$ | | | | | 137* | 42* | | | Hi-vol | $n$ | | | | | 313 | 321 | 81* | |
| | | | | | $\bar{x}$ | | | | | 17* | 22* | | | | $\bar{x}$ | | | | | 143 | 150 | 104* | |
| | | | | | $P_{98}$ | | | | | 86* | 55* | | | | $P_{98}$ | | | | | 372 | 371 | 233* | |
| | | | | | max | | | | | 94* | 68* | | | | max | | | | | 632 | 453 | 265* | |
| | | 12 | CCC | TCM | $n$ | | | | 216 | 173 | | | | Hi-vol | $n$ | | | | 350 | 316 | 314 | 307 | 290 |
| | | | | | $\bar{x}$ | | | | 6 | 17 | | | | | $\bar{x}$ | | | | 92 | 91 | 99 | 85 | 95 |
| | | | | | $P_{98}$ | | | | 13 | 55 | | | | | $P_{98}$ | | | | 189 | 178 | 200 | 168 | 175 |
| | | | | | max | | | | 52 | 92 | | | | | max | | | | 268 | 316 | 247 | 204 | 200 |
| | | 23 | CCI | | | | | | | | | | | Hi-vol | $n$ | | | | | | | 213 | 290 |
| | | | | | | | | | | | | | | | $\bar{x}$ | | | | | | | 65 | 63 |
| | | | | | | | | | | | | | | | $P_{98}$ | | | | | | | 284 | 282 |
| | | | | | | | | | | | | | | | max | | | | | | | 409 | 334 |
| | Fairfield, AL | 3 | SI | Coul | $n$ | | | | 268 | | | | | Hi-vol | $n$ | | | | 340 | 279 | 272 | 267 | 289 |
| | | | | | $\bar{x}$ | | | | 32 | | | | | | $\bar{x}$ | | | | 84 | 81 | 83 | 72 | 79 |
| | | | | | $P_{98}$ | | | | 110 | | | | | | $P_{98}$ | | | | 168 | 162 | 164 | 129 | 150 |
| | | | | | max | | | | 262 | | | | | | max | | | | 200 | 209 | 242 | 142 | 216 |
| | Azusa, CA | 2 | SI | Cond | $n$ | | | | 361 | | 271* | | | Hi-vol | $n$ | | | | 61* | 46* | 193* | | |
| | | | | | $\bar{x}$ | | | | 27 | | 19* | | | | $\bar{x}$ | | | | 108* | 148* | 174* | | |
| | | | | | $P_{98}$ | | | | 65 | | 55* | | | | $P_{98}$ | | | | 193* | 332* | 342* | | |
| | | | | | max | | | | 102 | | 69* | | | | max | | | | 226* | 430* | 477* | | |
| | Long Beach, CA | 1 | CCC | | | | | | | | | | | Hi-vol | $n$ | | | | 55 | 52 | 11* | | |
| | | | | | | | | | | | | | | | $\bar{x}$ | | | | 90 | 96 | 66* | | |
| | | | | | | | | | | | | | | | $P_{98}$ | | | | 192 | 171 | 105* | | |
| | | | | | | | | | | | | | | | max | | | | 218 | 180 | 105* | | |
| | Pasadena, CA | 2 | CCR | | | | | | | | | | | Hi-vol | $n$ | | | | 59 | 59 | | | |
| | | | | | | | | | | | | | | | $\bar{x}$ | | | | 74 | 88 | | | |
| | | | | | | | | | | | | | | | $P_{98}$ | | | | 131 | 168 | | | |
| | | | | | | | | | | | | | | | max | | | | 140 | 227 | | | |
| | | 4 | CCC | Cond | $n$ | | | | 364 | | 273 | | | Hi-vol | $n$ | | | | 61 | 45 | 50 | | |
| | | | | | $\bar{x}$ | | | | 38 | | 40 | | | | $\bar{x}$ | | | | 102 | 124 | 102 | | |
| | | | | | $P_{98}$ | | | | 68 | | 67 | | | | $P_{98}$ | | | | 178 | 230 | 189 | | |
| | | | | | max | | | | 97 | | 74 | | | | max | | | | 202 | 169 | 203 | | |

Annex 4 (*cont.*)

| Country | City | Site No. | Site Area | $SO_2$ Method | | $SO_2$ 73 | 74 | 75 | 76 | 77 | 78 | 79 | 80 | SPM Method | | SPM 73 | 74 | 75 | 76 | 77 | 78 | 79 | 80 |
|---|---|---|---|---|---|---|---|---|---|---|---|---|---|---|---|---|---|---|---|---|---|---|---|
| United States of America (*cont.*) | Chicago, IL | 3 | SR | | | | | | | | | | | Hi-vol | $n$ | | | | 117 | 100 | 113 | | |
| | | | | | | | | | | | | | | | $\bar{x}$ | | | | 68 | 83 | 70 | | |
| | | | | | | | | | | | | | | | $P_{98}$ | | | | 148 | 219 | 200 | | |
| | | | | | | | | | | | | | | | max | | | | 259 | 276 | 230 | | |
| | | 5 | CCC | | | | | | | | | | | Hi-vol | $n$ | | | | | 111 | 116 | | |
| | | | | | | | | | | | | | | | $\bar{x}$ | | | | | 86 | 87 | | |
| | | | | | | | | | | | | | | | $P_{98}$ | | | | | 183 | 189 | | |
| | | | | | | | | | | | | | | | max | | | | | 225 | 214 | | |
| | | 22 | CCI | TCM | $n$ | | | | 63 | 25* | | | | Hi-vol | $n$ | | | | 119 | 114 | 88 | 84 | 52 |
| | | | | | $\bar{x}$ | | | | 20 | 40* | | | | | $\bar{x}$ | | | | 146 | 200 | 136 | 138 | 129 |
| | | | | | $P_{98}$ | | | | 100 | 129* | | | | | $P_{98}$ | | | | 342 | 617 | 253 | 287 | 226 |
| | | | | | max | | | | 105 | 129* | | | | | max | | | | 474 | 1106 | 517 | 325 | 231 |
| | | 39 | CCI | Coul. | $n$ | | | | | | | 352 | 182* | | | | | | | | | | |
| | | | | | $\bar{x}$ | | | | | | | 48 | 37* | | | | | | | | | | |
| | | | | | $P_{98}$ | | | | | | | 173 | 107* | | | | | | | | | | |
| | | | | | max | | | | | | | 247 | 151* | | | | | | | | | | |
| | St Ann, MO | 1 | SC | FPD | $n$ | | | | 234 | 294 | 297 | | | Hi-vol | $n$ | | | | 49 | 53 | 56 | | |
| | | | | | $\bar{x}$ | | | | 32 | 308 | 36 | | | | $\bar{x}$ | | | | 65 | 64 | 65 | | |
| | | | | | $P_{98}$ | | | | 131 | 1022 | 147 | | | | $P_{98}$ | | | | 153 | 147 | 117 | | |
| | | | | | max | | | | 210 | 1362 | 210 | | | | max | | | | 172 | 167 | 138 | | |
| | St Charles, MO | 2 | SR | PFA | $n$ | | | | 202* | 143* | | | | Hi-vol | $n$ | | | | | 25* | | | |
| | | | | | $\bar{x}$ | | | | 14* | 10* | | | | | $\bar{x}$ | | | | | 66* | | | |
| | | | | | $P_{98}$ | | | | 67* | 69* | | | | | $P_{98}$ | | | | | 138* | | | |
| | | | | | max | | | | 191* | 151* | | | | | max | | | | | 138* | | | |

| Country | City | No. | Site | Method | Statistic | | | | | | | | | Method | Statistic | | | | | | | | |
|---|---|---|---|---|---|---|---|---|---|---|---|---|---|---|---|---|---|---|---|---|---|---|---|
| United States of America (*cont.*) | St Louis, MO | 1 | CCC | PFA | *n*<br>x̄<br>$P_{98}$<br>max | | | | | 263<br>101<br>529<br>700 | 341<br>30<br>87<br>200 | 291<br>31<br>105<br>142 | 316<br>37<br>95<br>238 | Hi-vol | *n*<br>x̄<br>$P_{98}$<br>max | 78<br>88<br>160<br>188 | 107<br>87<br>179<br>189 | 94<br>86<br>155<br>164 | | 118<br>96<br>237<br>420 | 83<br>99<br>191<br>913 | | |
| | | 3 | CCR | PFA | *n*<br>x̄<br>$P_{98}$<br>max | | | | | | | 355<br>50<br>148<br>218 | 354<br>59<br>151<br>215 | Hi-vol | *n*<br>x̄<br>$P_{98}$<br>max | 59<br>112<br>217<br>227 | 58<br>122<br>279<br>327 | 58<br>115<br>181<br>205 | | | | | |
| | | 4 | CCI | PFA | *n*<br>x̄<br>$P_{98}$<br>max | | | | | 199<br>104<br>529<br>700 | | 272*<br>21*<br>71*<br>96* | 349<br>25<br>88<br>153 | Hi-vol | *n*<br>x̄<br>$P_{98}$<br>max | 55<br>127<br>236<br>276 | 102<br>144<br>337<br>382 | 97<br>123<br>323<br>568 | 99<br>129<br>360<br>581 | 96<br>111<br>315<br>420 | | | |
| | | | | TCM | *n*<br>x̄<br>$P_{98}$<br>max | | | | 266<br>149<br>812<br>996 | 40*<br>166*<br>634*<br>700* | | | | | | | | | | | | | |
| | New York City, NY | 4 | SR | PFA | *n*<br>x̄<br>$P_{98}$<br>max | | | | | | 155*<br>49*<br>147*<br>214* | 364<br>48<br>122<br>204 | 365<br>43<br>136<br>229 | Hi-vol | *n*<br>x̄<br>$P_{98}$<br>max | | | | 137<br>60<br>149<br>177 | 86<br>64<br>127<br>149 | 18*<br>48*<br>94*<br>94* | 36*<br>49*<br>93*<br>94* | 56<br>51<br>96<br>100 |
| | | 10 | CCR | PFA | *n*<br>x̄<br>$P_{98}$<br>max | | | | | | 169*<br>72*<br>162*<br>269* | 339<br>80<br>212<br>292 | 362<br>75<br>191<br>312 | Hi-vol | *n*<br>x̄<br>$P_{98}$<br>max | | | | 95<br>77<br>150<br>178 | 110<br>79<br>146<br>153 | 25*<br>64*<br>117*<br>117* | 53<br>66<br>112<br>123 | 50<br>62<br>123<br>129 |
| | | 11 | CCI | PFA | *n*<br>x̄<br>$P_{98}$<br>max | | | | | | 59*<br>88*<br>203*<br>204* | 362<br>56<br>130<br>160 | 364<br>52<br>112<br>147 | Hi-vol | *n*<br>x̄<br>$P_{98}$<br>max | | | | | 94*<br>78*<br>131*<br>158* | 23*<br>68*<br>121*<br>121* | 59<br>64<br>121<br>126 | 53<br>63<br>109<br>124 |
| | Harris, TX | 24 | SR | PFA | *n*<br>x̄<br>$P_{98}$<br>max | | | | | | | 65*<br>10*<br>33*<br>35* | 132*<br>8*<br>35*<br>52* | Hi-vol | *n*<br>x̄<br>$P_{98}$<br>max | | | | 54<br>70<br>118<br>134 | 50<br>100<br>210<br>1041 | 50<br>80<br>133<br>151 | 19*<br>62*<br>144*<br>144* | 22*<br>64*<br>140*<br>140* |
| | | | | TCM | *n*<br>x̄<br>$P_{98}$<br>max | | | | 47<br>3<br>10<br>13 | 52<br>3<br>15<br>19 | 25<br>10<br>33<br>33 | | | | | | | | | | | | |

Annex 4 (*cont.*)

| Country | City | Site No. | Site Area | SO2 Method | | SO2 73 | SO2 74 | SO2 75 | SO2 76 | SO2 77 | SO2 78 | SO2 79 | SO2 80 | SPM Method | | SPM 73 | SPM 74 | SPM 75 | SPM 76 | SPM 77 | SPM 78 | SPM 79 | SPM 80 |
|---|---|---|---|---|---|---|---|---|---|---|---|---|---|---|---|---|---|---|---|---|---|---|---|
| United States of America (*cont.*) | Houston, TX | 1 | CCC | TCM | *n* | | | | | 41 | 57 | 19* | | Hi-vol | *n* | | | | | 39 | 47 | 51 | 52 |
| | | | | | x̄ | | | | | 4 | 16 | 14* | | | x̄ | | | | | 115 | 98 | 89 | 82 |
| | | | | | $P_{98}$ | | | | | 23 | 109 | 37* | | | $P_{98}$ | | | | | 300 | 192 | 147 | 142 |
| | | | | | max | | | | | 38 | 141 | 37* | | | max | | | | | 1333 | 209 | 158 | 156 |
| | | 34 | SR | PFA | *n* | | | | | | | 59* | 318 | | *n* | | | | 58 | 60 | 53 | 31* | 31* |
| | | | | | x̄ | | | | | | | 22* | 20 | | x̄ | | | | 95 | 113 | 106 | 91* | 97* |
| | | | | | $P_{98}$ | | | | | | | 69* | 86 | | $P_{98}$ | | | | 162 | 297 | 202 | 159* | 152* |
| | | | | | max | | | | | | | 98* | 108 | | max | | | | 198 | 842 | 206 | 166* | 152* |
| | | | | TCM | *n* | | | | 56 | 55 | 42 | 21* | | | | | | | | | | | |
| | | | | | x̄ | | | | 3 | 7 | 14 | 22* | | | | | | | | | | | |
| | | | | | $P_{98}$ | | | | 16 | 34 | 32 | 49* | | | | | | | | | | | |
| | | | | | max | | | | 21 | 42 | 149 | 49* | | | | | | | | | | | |
| Venezuela | Caracas | 1 | CCR | Acid | *n* | | | | 238 | 312 | | | | Smoke | *n* | | | | 238 | 313 | | | |
| | | | | | x̄ | | | | 7 | 9 | | | | | x̄ | | | | 20 | 23 | | | |
| | | | | | $P_{98}$ | | | | 14 | 21 | | | | | $P_{98}$ | | | | 39 | 44 | | | |
| | | | | | max | | | | 20 | 26 | | | | | max | | | | 58 | 49 | | | |
| | | 2 | CCC | Acid | *n* | | | | 302 | 226 | 61* | | | Smoke | *n* | | | | 310 | 226 | 61* | | |
| | | | | | x̄ | | | | 24 | 16 | 21* | | | | x̄ | | | | 31 | 28 | 25* | | |
| | | | | | $P_{98}$ | | | | 37 | 33 | 27* | | | | $P_{98}$ | | | | 56 | 52 | 39* | | |
| | | | | | max | | | | 40 | 42 | 31* | | | | max | | | | 62 | 79 | 43* | | |
| | | 3 | SI | Acid | *n* | | | | 248 | 231 | | | | Smoke | *n* | | | | 224 | 231 | | | |
| | | | | | x̄ | | | | 12 | 16 | | | | | x̄ | | | | 14 | 16 | | | |
| | | | | | $P_{98}$ | | | | 22 | 42 | | | | | $P_{98}$ | | | | 32 | 31 | | | |
| | | | | | max | | | | 28 | 44 | | | | | max | | | | 36 | 37 | | | |
| Yugoslavia | Zagreb | 1 | CCC | Acid | *n* | 307 | 354 | 354 | 363 | 364 | 317 | 351 | 323 | Membrane grav sampler | *n* | 202 | 213 | 205 | 206 | 151* | 176 | 174 | 197 |
| | | | | | x̄ | 195 | 158 | 144 | 142 | 115 | 112 | 81 | 94 | | x̄ | 181 | 167 | 179 | 170 | 163* | 171 | 135 | 180 |
| | | | | | $P_{98}$ | 595 | 511 | 492 | 494 | 400 | 402 | 282 | 257 | | $P_{98}$ | 512 | 452 | 417 | 383 | 362* | 342 | 436 | 320 |
| | | | | | max | 723 | 818 | 703 | 730 | 740 | 488 | 518 | 362 | | max | 611 | 806 | 486 | 621 | 450* | 452 | 587 | 830 |
| | | 2 | SR | Acid | *n* | 296 | 347 | 364 | 364 | 357 | 362 | 362 | 365 | Membrane grav sampler | *n* | 196 | 195 | 202 | 198 | 177 | 182 | 192 | 201 |
| | | | | | x̄ | 66 | 54 | 53 | 51 | 48 | 44 | 33 | 46 | | x̄ | 144 | 129 | 130 | 127 | 131 | 143 | 136 | 142 |
| | | | | | $P_{98}$ | 212 | 252 | 226 | 228 | 199 | 180 | 173 | 147 | | $P_{98}$ | 396 | 346 | 306 | 288 | 332 | 375 | 289 | 339 |
| | | | | | max | 381 | 456 | 364 | 388 | 296 | 363 | 407 | 290 | | max | 596 | 374 | 483 | 316 | 386 | 437 | 350 | 488 |
| | | 3 | CCI | Acid | *n* | 301 | 356 | 364 | 366 | 355 | 365 | 365 | 366 | Membrane grav sampler | *n* | 233 | 232 | 251 | 249 | 227 | 219 | 197 | 232 |
| | | | | | x̄ | 76 | 73 | 65 | 68 | 62 | 54 | 40 | 33 | | x̄ | 168 | 168 | 153 | 141 | 161 | 148 | 150 | 133 |
| | | | | | $P_{98}$ | 261 | 284 | 246 | 261 | 268 | 258 | 219 | 158 | | $P_{98}$ | 378 | 425 | 340 | 283 | 308 | 310 | 408 | 355 |
| | | | | | max | 353 | 420 | 428 | 506 | 426 | 347 | 365 | 280 | | max | 517 | 719 | 445 | 579 | 418 | 506 | 498 | 571 |